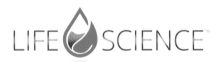

LIFE SCIENCE

Copyright © 2016
Life Science Publishing
1.800.336.6308
www.DiscoverLSP.com

Printed in the United States of America
10 9 8 7 6 5 4 3 2 1

TABLE OF CONTENTS

WELCOME TO ESSENTIAL OILS

Perhaps you have experienced essential oils in the past, perhaps in a spa treatment or in body care products. The aromatic properties of these essential oils are just a small part of their incredible story. The world of essential oils opens the door to health-promoting botanicals that can be diffused, inhaled, applied topically, incorporated into massage or taken internally, all to support your health and wellness. The oils listed within these pages are not a complete list of every oil you can use to combat each ailment.

For a complete list of oils and their possible uses, please reference the *Essential Oil Desk Reference, Quick Reference Guide* and *Pocket Reference Guide.*

PROMOTE A HEALTHY EMOTIONAL STATE

Each essential oil boasts a complex, pleasant, and unique scent that will activate the brain's center of emotion and memory (the limbic system) in a different way. Some essential oils may uplift the spirits. Others help you release negative thoughts and habits. They can be your key to a more fulfilling and balanced emotional life.

You can use the following oils and blends for diffusion, soothing baths, massage, inhalation, or topical application to help you rediscover peace, balance, and joy:

- Joy™
- Orange
- Peppermint
- Lavender
- Peace & Calming™
- Jasmine

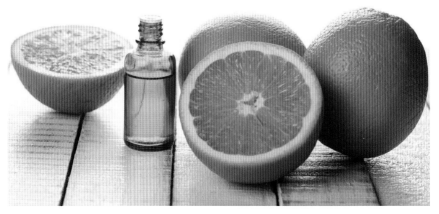

IMPROVE YOUR PHYSICAL WELLNESS

Life gets busier and more chaotic each day, and your lifestyle doesn't always create an ideal opportunity to maintain physical wellness. Poor diet, lack of exercise and being pummeled by environmental toxins can leave the body unbalanced. From cleansing and weight management to supporting all of the systems in your body, essential oils and essential oil-infused supplements can provide the solutions you need.

Feel alive and refreshed every day with nutrients, powerful antioxidants, and pure essential oils found in these products:

- · NingXia Red™
- · Life 5™
- · Slique™ Tea
- · OmegaGize3™
- · Longevity™

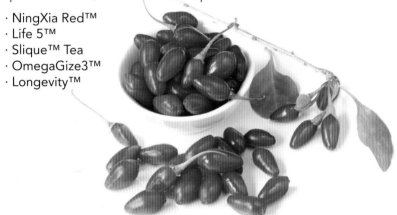

CLEANSE YOUR HOME AND SURROUNDINGS

You don't have to use harsh chemicals to clean your home. You can polish countertops, remove sticky messes, repel bugs and clean dirty areas with the gentle and effective power of essential oils and Thieves™ products.

There are convenient and non-chemical options for cleaning your home, leaving only pleasant scents and a healthy environment. You can replace most cleansers with versatile products, such as:

- · Thieves Household Cleaner®
- · Lemon Essential Oil
- · Purification Essential Oil
- · Thyme Essential Oil
- · Lemongrass Essential Oil

REFINE YOUR SKIN

Rediscover your natural glow and purge chemicals from your beauty routine. Essential Oils can help soothe tension, support healthy cell growth, promote a clear complexion, soften signs of aging, and nurture healthy hair.

- · A·R·T® Renewal Serum
- · Boswellia Wrinkle Cream
- · Frankincense
- · Lavender Volume Shampoo/Conditioner
- · Copaiba Vanilla Shampoo/Conditioner

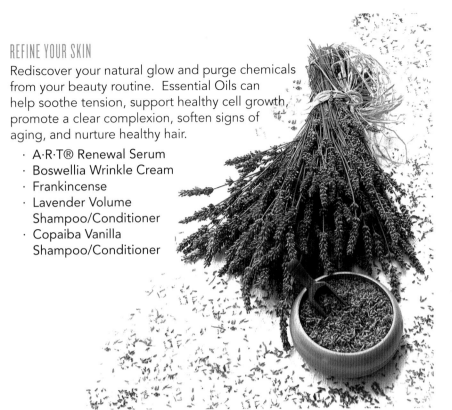

PROMOTE SPIRITUAL AWARENESS

Incense and essential oils from plants have always had a starring role in religious and spiritual ceremonies, helping those involved to transcend the trivial and connect with something larger than themselves.

To enhance your spiritual experience, dilute and apply meditative, empowering essential oils directly to wrists, feet, and behind the ears, or diffuse in a quiet area. Popular oils and blends for spiritual focus include:

- · Sacred Frankincense
- · White Angelica™
- · Egyptian Gold™
- · Inspiration™
- · The Gift™

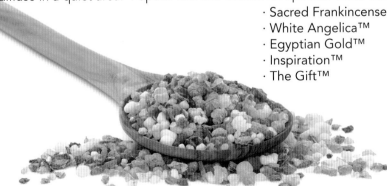

ALLERGIES

Allergies are a result of the response to many different situations. They can be triggered by food, pollen, environmental chemicals, pet dander, dust, insect bites, to name just a few, and can affect the following:

- Respiration—wheezing, labored breathing
- Mouth—swelling of the lips or tongue, itching lips
- Digestive tract—diarrhea, vomiting, cramps
- Skin—rashes, dermatitis
- Nose—sneezing, congestion, bloody nose

Food allergies are different from food intolerances. Food allergies involve an immune system reaction, whereas food intolerances involve gastrointestinal reactions and are far more common.

For example, peanuts often produce a lifelong allergy due to peanut proteins being targeted by immune system antibodies as foreign invaders. In contrast, intolerance of pasteurized cow's milk that causes cramping and diarrhea is due to the inability to digest lactose (milk sugar) because of a lack of the enzyme lactase.

Food allergies are often associated with the consumption of peanuts, shellfish, nuts, wheat, cow's milk, eggs, and soy. Infants and children are far more prone to have food allergies than adults, due to the immaturity of their immune and digestive systems.

WHAT YOU WILL NEED...

Oil Blends	Single Oils	Also try...
• Breathe Again Roll-on™	• Lavender	• NingXia Red
• Tranquil Roll-on™	• Roman Chamomile	
• R.C.™		

Allergies can be caused by hay fever, seasonal changes, poison ivy, poison oak, plants, molds, foods, animals, insect bites, drugs, cosmetics & cleaners.

It is a common misconception that allergies are chronic and impossible to escape. By addressing the issue at the source, you may be able to improve your chances. Take a proactive approach and start using your favorite oils at least one month before allergies normally strike. This may help to reduce the length and severity of your allergy season.

MAY WE ALSO SUGGEST...

TOPICAL:
Apply Breathe Again Roll-on
along both sides of the nose, on
the back of the neck, and down
the throat. This may help relieve
allergy symptoms. Tranquil Roll-
on, when applied around the areas
of a rash, may soothe the itch.

DIFFUSING:
Use Lavender at night and RC during the
day to support normal respiration.

ADDITIONAL USES:
Drink approximately 1 oz of NingXia Red with
1 full capsule of Lavender 2-4 times a day.
If symptoms persist, add 2 drops of Roman
Chamomile to the Lavender capsule.

ASTHMA

During an asthma attack, the bronchial air tubes in the lungs become swollen and clogged with thick, sticky mucus. The muscles of the air tubes will also begin to constrict or tighten. This results in very difficult or labored breathing. If an attack is severe, it can actually be life-threatening. Many asthma attacks are triggered by an allergic reaction to pollen, skin particles, dandruff, cat and dog dander, dust mites, as well as from foods such as eggs, milk, flavorings, dyes, preservatives, and other chemicals. Asthma can also be triggered by respiratory infection, exercise, stress, and psychological factors.

If you are prone to asthma, practice your relaxation techniques and be prepared. Carry Stress Away Roll-on™ and apply Peace & Calming™, Tranquil Roll-on or RutaVaLa™ to your feet each night to help fortify your body against an asthma attack and improve your balance. You can be proactive by applying the oils when your asthma is under control.

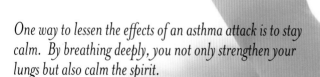

One way to lessen the effects of an asthma attack is to stay calm. By breathing deeply, you not only strengthen your lungs but also calm the spirit.

Asthma affects more than 17 million people in the United States and more than one-third of those affected are children.

TOPICAL:

Apply Breathe Again Roll-On and Eucalyptus Blue™ to your chest, back, and the bottom of your feet twice a day (morning and night). Apply 1-2 drops of Ortho Ease™, Relaxation™, or Sensation™ massage oils on your temples and the back of your neck. You can also apply 2-3 drops on the Vita Flex™ points on your feet.

DIFFUSING:

Establish rotation between 3 oils: R.C., Raven™ & Hyssop - approximately 15 minutes per day to support healthy respiration. Seek medical attention if you are experiencing an asthma attack!

ADDITIONAL USES:

Add 2 drops of Frankincense and 2 drops of Lemon to 1 ounce of NingXia Red, 2-4 times a day.

WHAT YOU WILL NEED...

Oil Blends
- Breathe Again Roll-on
- Peace & Calming
- Raven
- RC
- RutaVaLa Roll-on
- Tranquil Roll-on

Single Oils
- Eucalyptus Blue
- Frankincense
- Hyssop
- Lavender
- Lemon

Also try...
- NingXia Red

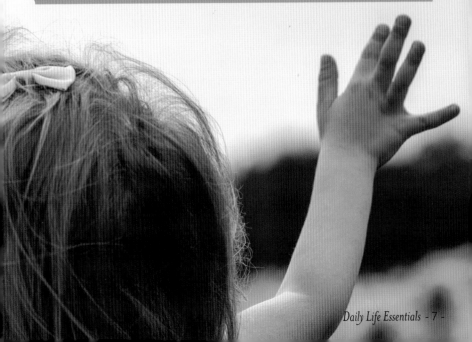

AUTISM

Autism is one of the concerns that can affect the brain. It is a neurologically based developmental disorder that is four times more common in boys than in girls. It can be characterized by

- Social Ineptness
- Nonverbal and Verbal Communication Difficulties
- Repetitive Behavior (rocking, hair twirling, etc.)
- Self-injurious Behavior (head banging)
- Very Limiting or Peculiar Interests
- Reduced or Abnormal Responses to Pain, Noises or other Outside Stimuli

Some researchers believe that gastrointestinal disorders may be linked to the brain dysfunction that can cause autism. Stimulating the limbic region of the brain may also help treat the symptoms of autism.

Improving your diet can be the key to reducing problems associated with autism; for example, try exchanging refined and synthetic sugars with natural sweeteners such as agave, natural fruit sweeteners, and 100% real maple syrup. You may also consider taking enzymes before meals in an effort to improve symptoms such as attention deficit, socialization, hyperactivity, eye contact, compulsions and comprehension.

MAY WE ALSO SUGGEST...

TOPICAL:
Apply 1-2 drops (undiluted) on temples and back of neck as desired. A single drop under your nose is also helpful and refreshing. Massage 2-4 drops of oil (neat) on the soles of the feet just before bedtime - kids love it!

DIFFUSING:
For 30 minutes every 4-6 hours you can diffuse your choice of oils. You may also choose to place 2-3 drops of your chosen oil in your hands and rub them together; inhale throughout the day.

ADDITIONAL USES:
Special Recipe: 15 Drops Frankincense, 12 Drops Myrrh, 10 Drops Idaho Balsam Fir, 4 drops Peppermint (take 1 capsule 3 times daily)

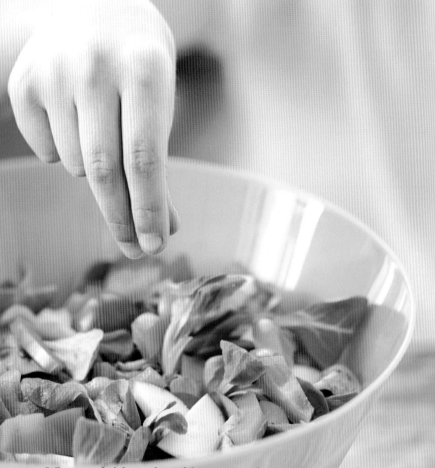

WHAT YOU WILL NEED...

Oil Blends
- Brain Power™
- Valor™ (and roll-on)
- Clarity™
- Peace & Calming
- Common Sense™
- The Gift

Single Oils
- Vetiver
- Patchouli
- Lavender
- Eucalyptus
- Melissa
- Cedarwood
- Sandalwood
- Frankincense

Also try...
- NingXia Red
- Power Meal™
- Balance Complete™

When you feel foggy, forgetful, or scattered, it may be time to feed your brain. The brain is made up of mostly fat, and will perform at its highest level when we feed it. Our brain not only controls how we think but also how the rest of our body's systems perform.

BRAIN POWER

Attention deficit hyperactivity disorder (ADHD) and attention deficit disorder (ADD) symptoms may begin in childhood and continue into adulthood. ADHD and ADD symptoms, such as hyperactivity, impulsiveness and inattentiveness, can cause problems at home, school, work, or in relationships. Terry Friedmann, MD, in 2001 completed pioneering studies using essential oils to combat ADD and ADHD. By inhaling essential oils including Vetiver, Cedarwood, and Lavender twice a day, Dr. Friedmann was able to show significant results in 60 days. Essential oils can stimulate the limbic system of the brain which may help mitigate ADD and ADHD. Attention disorders may be caused by mineral deficiencies in the diet, so increasing nutrient intake and absorption of magnesium, potassium, and other trace minerals can also have a beneficial effect.

Dr. Friedmann's studies also showed that the aroma from therapeutic essential oils have an amazing ability to stimulate the limbic region of the brain. The sense of smell is tied directly to the mind's emotional and hormonal centers and this connection has the potential to exert a powerful influence on ADD/ADHD and autism.

MAY WE ALSO SUGGEST...

TOPICAL:
Apply a few drops of Brain Power to the big toes and Sacred Frankincense, Valor, Stress Away Roll-on, and RutaVaLa Roll-on to the spine. Additionally, apply Helichrysum to the brain stem to support the central nervous system.

DIFFUSING:
Use Cedarwood day and night. You can also add Lavender or Peace & Calming to help you sleep more soundly.

ADDITIONAL USES:
Take Omega Blue & Longevity capsules 1-2 times daily.
Take 1-2 SleepEssence Capsules at night to help with sleeping.

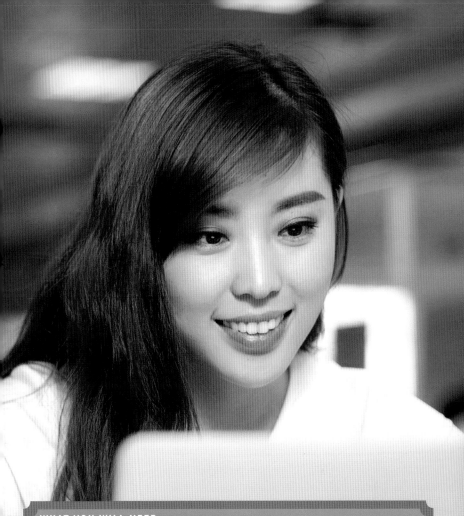

WHAT YOU WILL NEED...

Oil Blends
- Brain Power
- Valor
- Clarity
- Peace & Calming
- RutaVaLa
- Stress Away Roll-On

Single Oils
- Lavender
- Cedarwood
- Sandalwood
- Cardamom
- Peppermint
- Frankincense

Also try...
- NingXia Red
- OmegaGize³
- SleepEssence™

Students who study late at night and use caffeine to stay awake often find that their short-term memory fails them the next day.

Studies show that you can skip the coffee or soda and instead, take a shot or two of NingXia Red and 4 Multigreens capsules to have much better memory performance. You can repeat this regimen every four hours.

BREAST HEALTH

You are the first line of defense for the health of your breasts! By conducting self-exams on your breasts regularly, you can become familiar with them and easily notice even the smallest of changes. Gary Young has developed a program to promote breast health and you can engage in that program twice a year - the national Breast Cancer Awareness months are in April and October. Frankincense, Tsuga™, Myrtle and Sandalwood may be applied to the breasts every day for the entire month (dilute with a delivery oil if you experience any discomfort).

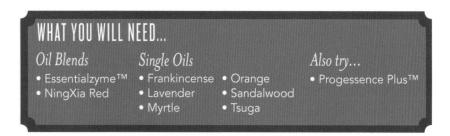

WHAT YOU WILL NEED...

Oil Blends
- Essentialzyme™
- NingXia Red

Single Oils
- Frankincense
- Lavender
- Myrtle
- Orange
- Sandalwood
- Tsuga

Also try...
- Progessence Plus™

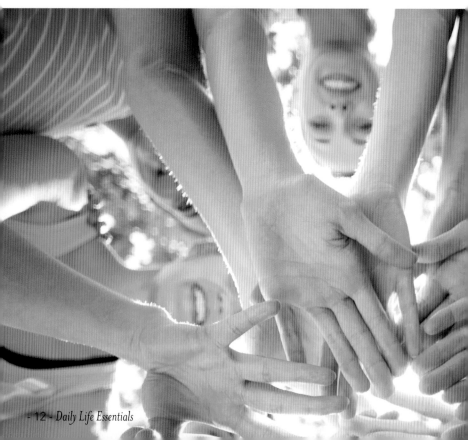

MAY WE ALSO SUGGEST...

TOPICAL:
Apply 1-4 drops of Frankincense daily to each breast and use 1-2 drops of Progessence Plus on any fatty tissue such as the hips, stomach and thighs.

DIFFUSING:
Use Lavender at night to promote healthy cell regeneration and encourage good sleep.

ADDITIONAL USES:
You can also drink 2 ounces of NingXia Red daily

Cancer feeds on sugar. Limiting your intake of sugars can significantly reduce your risk of breast cancers.
Stay familiar with your breasts. Changes in breast shape, size and feel can occur. This is common and most of them are benign. By conducting regular self-examinations and staying in close contact with your doctor about your breast health, you can detect problems as early as possible.

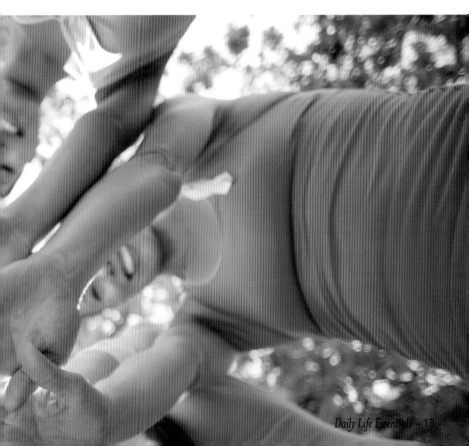

BUG BITES & REPELLENTS

Essential oils are ideal for treating most kinds of insect bites because of their amazing antiseptic and oil-soluble properties. Essential oils such as Lavender and Peppermint reduce insect-bite induced itching and infection.

Bug Bite Remedies: (apply 1-2 drops, neat or diluted 50/50 on location)
- 2 drops Thyme
- 10 drops Lavender
- 4 drops Eucalyptus
- 3 drops German Chamomile

Bug Specific:
- Black Widow Spider Bite - one drop of any oil including Purification, Melrose™, The Gift, Lemon then seek emergency care immediately
- Brown Recluse Spider Bite - 1 drop Lavender, 1 drop Myrrh, 1 drop Melrose - apply every 10 minutes until you reach professional medical assistance

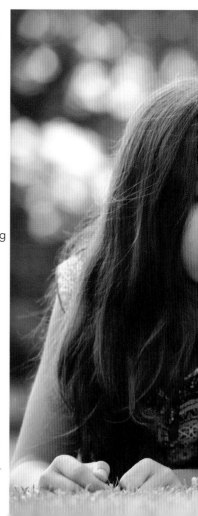

MAY WE ALSO SUGGEST...

TOPICAL:
Apply Purification to the bite to reduce swelling and draw out the poison. PanAway can be applied to the bite site to reduce pain and inflammation. Repeat until symptoms subside. Use the Bug Bite Remedy 2-4 times daily.

DIFFUSING:
Diffuse Purification to help keep bugs away from the area - they won't want to come back!

ADDITIONAL USES:
You may want to use Inner Defense every day for a week after being bitten. NingXia Red (1 oz) and Longevity (1 capsule) can help support your immune system.

WHAT YOU WILL NEED...

Oil Blends	Single Oils		Also try...
• PanAway™	• Peppermint	• Rosemary	• Inner Defense™
• Purification	• Lavender	• Copaiba	• Longevity™
• Tranquil Roll-on	• Citronella	• Dorado Azul	• NingXia Red
• Melrose	• Eucalyptus	• Melaleuca	

Even though every bite isn't necessarily toxic, insects can transmit diseases to you and to your pets.

Whenever possible, it is best to avoid areas infested with bugs. Toxic bites or not, it is still very uncomfortable. If you are unfortunate enough to be bitten, try to discover what kind of bug did it and, if necessary, have it tested.

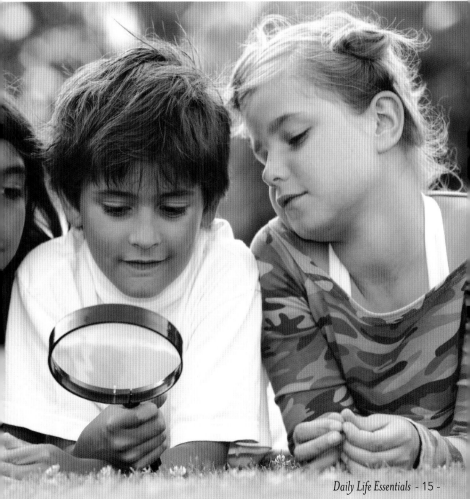

BURNS

There are three types of burns - first, second and third degree. First-degree burns only damage the outer later of skin; a sunburn is typically a First-degree burn. Second-degree burns damage the outer layer and move on to cause damage to the underlying later known as the dermis; this is usually manifested by blistering. Third-degree burns not only destroy or damage skin but can even cause damage to the underlying tissue.

Burns can be caused by the sun, chemicals, electricity, radiation and heat. Thermal burns (heat) are the most common type of burn. LavaDerm™ is used extensively in the treatment of burns and has been tested in being used as an anti-inflammatory and in promoting tissue regeneration.

Scars can develop on the skin's surface as the result of a burn, deep laceration or myriad of other injuries that break through the skin. The skin forms a scab over a wound within 3-4 days following an injury. By the tenth day, the scab will typically shrink and fall off because the body is focusing on another healing process, laying down collagen fibers to strengthen the wound site. In the case of a severe injury, this can take three months. Gently massage around the wound area to help promote healing and diminish scarring. Even just 15 minutes a day can make a noticeable difference in the healing process.

WHAT YOU WILL NEED...

Oil Blends	Single Oils		Also try...
• PanAway	• Clove	• Valerian	• NingXia Red
• Peace & Calming	• Cypress	• Vetiver	• OmegaGize[3]
• Melrose	• Frankincense	• Spikenard	• Sulfurzyme™
• Helichrysum	• Helichrysum	• Lavender	
• LavaDerm Spray	• Lavender	• G. Chamomile	
• Gentle Baby™			

Burns tend to swell and blister because of fluid loss from the damaged blood vessels. Staying hydrated after being burned is critical.

In the case of a serious burn, the victim can even go into shock, caused by severe fluid loss. This may require intravenous transfusions of saline to raise blood pressure and bring the body back to a healthy state. Seek medical attention for serious burns as needed.

► MAY WE ALSO SUGGEST...

TOPICAL:
Apply PanAway around the affected area (never put it directly on the wound). Apply Cypress to the feet to help with pain (not near the wound). Once a scab forms, you can apply Frankincense, Helichrysum, or Lavender to promote healing.

DIFFUSING:
Diffuse Peace & Calming to help you relax - you will heal faster if you're not worked up and tense.

ADDITIONAL USES:
Drink NingXia Red and take OmegaGize[3] and Sulfurzyme. Combine Clove, Helichrysum, Vetiver, and Valerian (2 drops each) in a capsule to help minimize the pain.

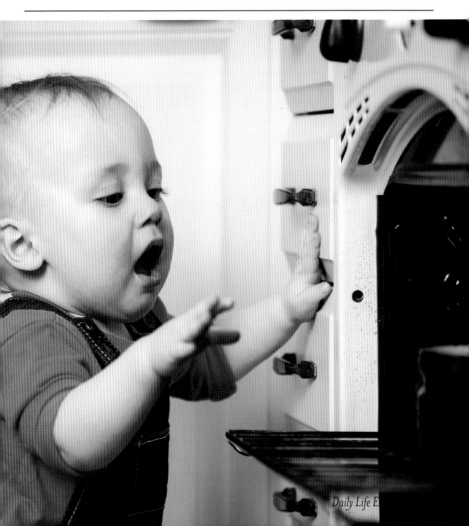

Daily Life E

CANDIDA AND YEAST INFECTION

Yeast and Candida are microorganisms that live in every human body. When your body is not in balance, problems can arise. There are many causes of that imbalance, including medications, diet, genetics, age, hydration, and more. The solution can vary from person to person, but keeping a healthy diet and maintaining good hygiene can support your body's balance. Medications and drugs can wipe out intestinal flora and provide an ideal environment for an overgrowth of yeast, including steroids and estrogen in the form of birth control or hormone replacement therapy.

Another manifestation of Candida is Thrush, most commonly found in babies. Thrush can develop very quickly, even overnight, and may become chronic and persist over a long period of time. A common indicator of Thrush is creamy white, slightly raised lesions in the mouth, usually on the tongue or inner cheek.

Vaginal yeast infections are usually caused from overgrowth of fungi, like Candida albicans. When excess sugar is consumed and when antibiotics are used, these organisms transform form harmless yeast into an invasive harmful fungus that secretes toxins as a part of its life cycle. Diet and cleansing are two major factors in overcoming this problem.

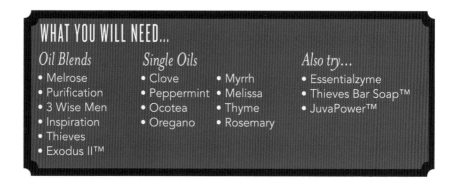

WHAT YOU WILL NEED...

Oil Blends
- Melrose
- Purification
- 3 Wise Men
- Inspiration
- Thieves
- Exodus II™

Single Oils
- Clove
- Peppermint
- Ocotea
- Oregano
- Myrrh
- Melissa
- Thyme
- Rosemary

Also try...
- Essentialzyme
- Thieves Bar Soap™
- JuvaPower™

Candida albicans is a naturally occurring yeast in the body. Yeast can grow out of control if the body's naturally check-and-balance system is out of whack.

Candida can thrive in warm, moist places on the body such as the mouth, vagina, or folds of the skin. By using Thieves Bar Soap or another topical soap, as well as a nutritional supplement and essential oil program, you can help maintain the body's balance, both inside and out.

TOPICAL:

Apply Melrose and Oregano to the bottoms of the feet. Oregano is an excellent oil for children too - always dilute it for children! By limiting their exposure to excess sugar and excess prescription medication, you can make huge strides in avoiding yeast overgrowth in their bodies.

DIFFUSING:

You can diffuse Peppermint to clear the mind and reduce cravings.

ADDITIONAL USES:

Try four drops of Ocotea under the tongue before meals, 1 drop of Clove on the tip of the tongue to reduce sugar cravings. Try Alkalyme™ and Life 5™(diluted 50:50) pro-biotic capsules to help promote an environment that doesn't encourage excessive yeast growth.

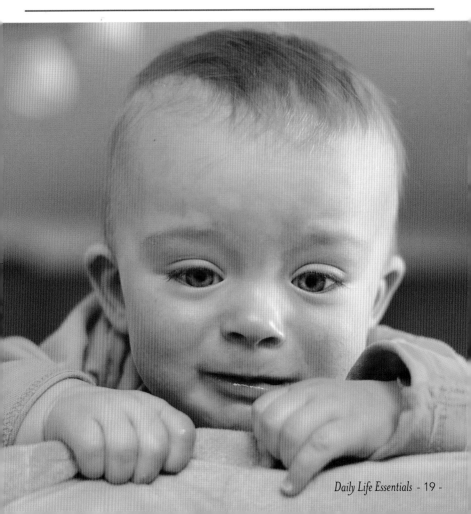

CLEANING

The market is flooded with cleaning products that contain chemicals that can often be harmful to you, your family and animals. Chemicals can linger for more than two weeks after you clean! As you use different cleaners, the chemicals in each one can mix into a toxic combination. Your family, friends and pets can be breathing harmful air. Commercial air fresheners can just contribute to the problem rather than removing these harmful toxins from your air. Thieves is an essential oil blend that includes Clove, Lemon, Cinnamon Bark, Eucalyptus, and Rosemary. Thieves™ is safe to touch, can be used on nearly any surface and doesn't leave a toxic residue behind.

Thieves Spray is an all natural, petrochemical-free antiseptic spray ideal for purifying small surfaces like doorknobs, handles, toilet seats and more. You can use it to spray any surface that needs cleansing and protection from dust, mold, and other microorganisms. The same powerful cleanser is available in Thieves Wipes™, Thieves Foaming Hand Soap™, and Thieves Waterless Hand Purifier™.

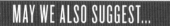

MAY WE ALSO SUGGEST...

TOPICAL:
Apply Thieves Cleaner to any surface - kitchen, bath, etc. Always test a small spot before cleaning the entire area. For tough stains and mold try a 50/50 dilution.

DIFFUSING:
You can diffuse oils every day - essential oils are used to fight airborne germs and odors. Try Thieves, Lemon, Grapefruit, Purification and Citrus Fresh.

ADDITIONAL USES:
When cleaning glass, add a cup of vinegar with one capful of Thieves Cleaner to a 32 oz spray bottle and fill with water.

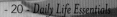

Essential Oils have been used for centuries to clean. They boast anti-pathogenic properties which can help keep your home, vehicle, and workplace clean and smelling fresh.

Just a few drops of essential oils go a long way when cleaning! You can add Melaleuca Alternifolia or Grapefruit to your Thieves cleaning solution, or add directly to your sponge, dish water, and the clothes dryer to fight odors and germs.

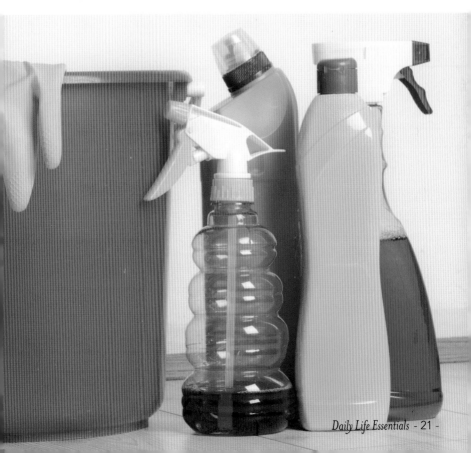

COLDS

One of the most effective ways to use essential oils to fight off a cold is to start using them when the first symptom strikes and then repeating. Using the oils in rotation can make a huge difference in how the cold will affect you and how long it will last. Ideally, you will use essential oils every 20 minutes. Another way to help prevent colds is by keeping your home and workspace clean and as free from germs as possible. By diffusing essential oils regularly you can help cleanse the air around you.

Although diffusing can be helpful, you may want to take a more direct approach by adding a few drops of oil to a bowl of boiling water, drape a towel over your head and the bowl to create a steam tent. With your eyes closed to avoid irritation, breathe deeply for 5-10 minutes and repeat this process 2-3 times while symptoms persist. Essential oils can help loosen mucus, and soothe the throat, nasal passages and bronchial tubes, specifically Thyme, Rosemary, Lemon and Thieves. Remember to drink plenty of water to stay hydrated!

MAY WE ALSO SUGGEST...

TOPICAL:
Apply Thieves, ImmuPower™, and Purification to the feet. Apply RC and Raven to the chest and back. Use Thieves cleaners to wipe down household surfaces including light switches, door knobs and phones.

DIFFUSING:
You can Thieves or Purification alternately all day.

ADDITIONAL USES:
Combine 2 ounces of NingXia Red with one Inner Defense capsule during the day. Combine 2 ounces of NingXia Red with one Life 5 capsule at night.

"Common Cold" is not just a clever name – colds are indeed common to us all and contribute to more lost work and school than any other illness.

Colds are typically caused by a virus and can last up to 21 days. Colds affect more than your physical health. While fighting a cold, you can begin to feel depressed, sad, and experience more fatigue than when you are healthy.

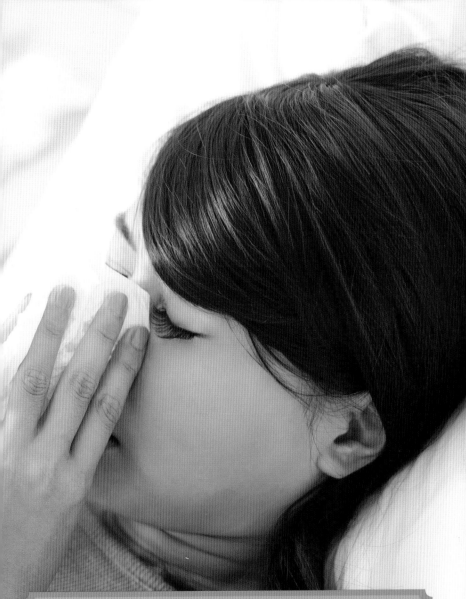

WHAT YOU WILL NEED...

Oil Blends
- ImmuPower
- Purification
- Raven
- RC
- Thieves

Single Oils
- Eucalyptus Radiata
- Lemon
- Rosemary
- Thyme

Also try...
- Inner Defense
- NingXia Red
- Thieves Cleaner

CONGESTION

Congestion can be one of the most painful and frustrating parts of the common cold. Your nasal pages can become blocked due to inflammation of the membranes lining the nose. As mucous accumulates in the chest, the blood vessels can become swollen.

In addition to inhaling and topically applying essential oils, you can also ingest them in an effort to fight off congestion. The amount of oil ingestion varies with different oils. Whether you put the oils in a capsule or drink them with a delivery liquid, you may want to start slowly at first to see how your body will react to a specific oil. Follow the guidelines and use common sense. Trust your body, focus on your intuitive feelings and what you have learned about using essential oils. No matter what you take, your body will benefit as long as you don't overdo it. So start slowly and be aware of your body's response.

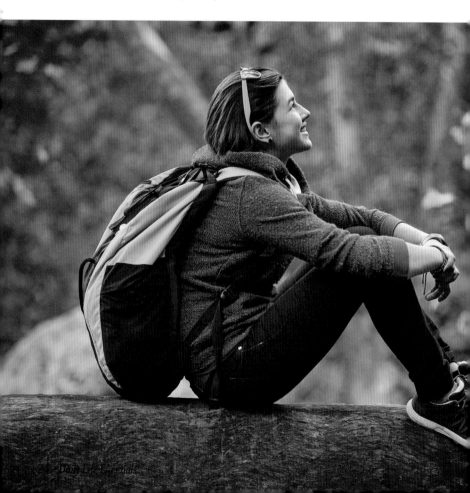

MAY WE ALSO SUGGEST...

TOPICAL:
You can use a warm compress with Frankincense, R.C., or Lavender over your chest and back. Apply Hyssop, Raven or Dorado Azul™ and cover with warm towel or blanket to maintain body temperature.

DIFFUSING:
Diffuse your choice of oils for 30 minutes every 4-6 hours or as desired. Try RC or Peppermint throughout the day.

ADDITIONAL USES:
Put 2-3 drops of your chosen oil in your hands, rub them together, cup your hands over your nose and inhale deeply. You can easily repeat throughout the day.

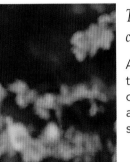

There are more natural and risk free ways to relieve congestion than commercial cold medicines.

Apply both Breathe Again and Tranquil Roll-ons to the sinuses on either side of your nose. This combination provides the power of a decongestant and an antihistamine without some of the negative side effects that a drug would cause.

WHAT YOU WILL NEED...

Oil Blends
- Breathe Again Roll-on
- Melrose
- Peace & Calming
- RC
- Raven
- Thieves
- Tranquil Roll-on

Single Oils
- Cedarwood
- Dorado Azul
- Eucalyptus
- Frankincense
- Goldenrod
- Ledum
- Marjoram
- Myrrh
- Peppermint
- Ravintsara

Also try...
- Inner Defense
- ImmuPro
- NingXia Red
- Super C™
- Thieves

CONSTIPATION

The primary causes of constipation are inadequate fluid intake and low fiber consumption. Constipation can eventually lead to diverticulosis and diverticulitis, most common among older people. By maintaining a healthy diet, you can avoid the discomfort of constipation and other more serious issues. Certain essential oils have also demonstrated their ability to help maintain a healthy colon by supporting intestinal flora, stimulating intestinal motility, fighting infections and eliminating parasites.

Don't be afraid to talk to your doctor about irregularity. If you develop hemorrhoids, apply a few drops of Melrose diluted with oil to the affected area to help ease pain and reduce swelling.

WHAT YOU WILL NEED...

Oil Blends
- DiGize™
- Juva Cleanse
- Melrose
- V-6™ Mixing Oil

Single Oils
- Anise Seed
- Fennel
- Ginger
- Peppermint
- Tangerine

Also try...
- Balance Complete™
- Comfortone®
- NingXia Red
- Life 5

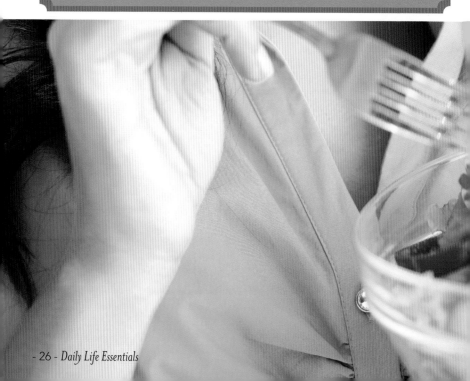

TOPICAL:

Apply a drop of DiGize, Peppermint or Ginger to a warm compress and place on your abdomen. Use the same oils on the shins and gently massage up and down your legs for ten minutes to stimulate digestion. You may want to dilute the essential oils when applying them to your shins to make massaging easier.

DIFFUSING:

Place 2-3 drops on a cotton ball and place it in an air vent in your home, car or work place.

ADDITIONAL USES:

Combine two ounces of NingXia Red with 3-4 drops of DiGize Vitality in a capsule during the day, and Comfortone capsules and a Life 5 capsule at night. Drink plenty of water to stay hydrated and avoid binding foods like white flour products, sugar, and chocolate.

Constipation is the general term we use for bowel movements that are infrequent and/or hard to pass.

Constipation can be caused by not getting enough fluids throughout the day but it may not be your fault. We have a tendency to lose the ability to feel thirst as we grow older. Establishing a routine of drinking water regularly throughout the day, whether you "feel" thirsty or not, can help alleviate constipation.

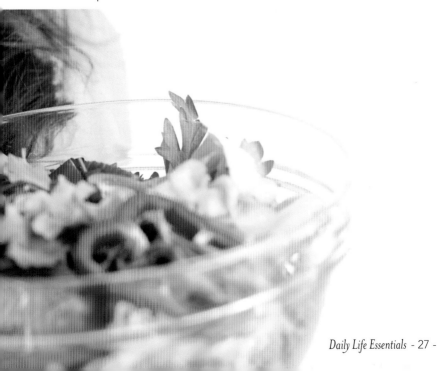

COUGH

To anyone who has ever had a cough, it is a common perception that nighttime brings on the worst of any cough. Especially as adults, a cough can last longer than it should because we don't get proper sleep and enough rest to allow our bodies to heal. Getting to sleep, and staying asleep, can make all the difference in how quickly we return to health. Try taking ImmuPro capsules at least 30 minutes before bed to help relax your body and support your natural immune system, in addition to the other oils you're taking for your cough and for sleep. Lavender and RC may be applied to the chest and back as well.

MAY WE ALSO SUGGEST...

TOPICAL:
Add drops of RC, Eucalyptus Globulus, Eucalyptus Blue, Frankincense or Lavender to a warm compress and place on chest and back. Follow with Hyssop, Dorado Azul or Raven.

DIFFUSING:
Diffuse R.C. or Peppermint on and off all day in the room where you are resting. You can easily make a small diffuser with a cup of boiling water and a couple of drops of essential oils - perfect for small spaces.

ADDITIONAL USES:
You may also choose to use Thieves Fresh Essence plus Mouthwash, Thieves Hard/Soft Lozenges, Thieves Spray

---

A cough can be highly painful and disruptive no matter what type it is.

Coughs can be dry, wet, or productive. Others are so intense that they can cause you to spasm. You may want to try 2 or 3 different oils before you find exactly the right combination for your particular cough.

WHAT YOU WILL NEED...

Oil Blends	Single Oils		Also try...
• Breathe Again™	• Dorado Azul	• Hyssop	• ImmuPro
• Raven	• Eucalyptus	• Lavender	• Inner Defense
• RC	Blue	• Lemon	• NingXia Red
• RutaVaLa Roll-on	• Eucalyptus	• Marjoram	
• Stress Away Roll-On	Globulus	• Peppermint	
• Thieves	• Frankincense		

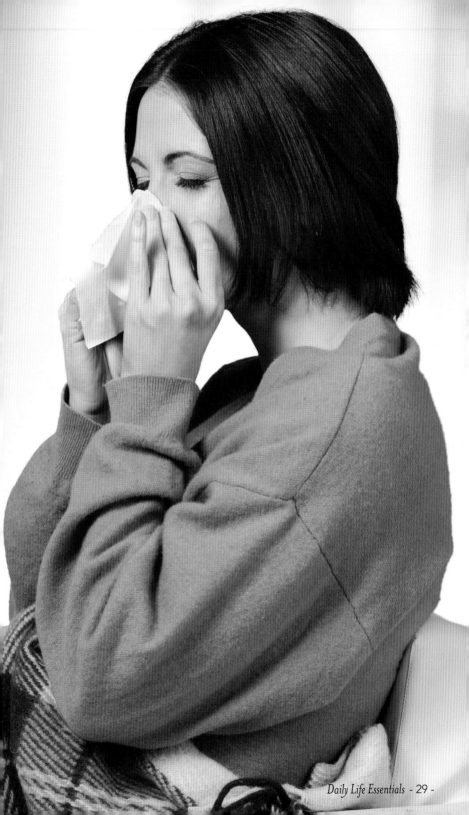

CUTS, SCRAPES, & BRUISES

Not all injuries result in a bruise, and those results vary with age. Small children may fall and get bumped more frequently but it can take quite a bit of force to bruise them. In an older person, minor bumps and scrapes can cause dramatic bruising. Blood vessels become more fragile with age and bruising can occur without injury in an elderly person. With any medication you are taking, ask questions about possible side effects including random bruising.

With minor cuts and scrapes, we often reach first for a triple antibiotic cream or something similar. This can be quite unnecessary and there may be a more simple option. Melaleuca Alternifolia can be applied straight to the skin and its natural properties can immediately support the healing process.

WHAT YOU WILL NEED...

Oil Blends
- Melrose
- Peace & Calming

Single Oils
- Frankincense
- Helichrysum
- Lavender
- Melaleuca Alternifolia

Also try...
- True Source™
- Super B™
- LavaDerm Spray

MAY WE ALSO SUGGEST...

TOPICAL:
Apply a clean, warm cloth to the injured area to clean it and remove debris. Lightly spritz Lavender Spray and apply Melrose topically. Cover as needed. Once the wound has fully closed, apply Lavender, Frankincense and Helichrysum to reduce scarring.

DIFFUSING:
Diffuse Peace & Calming to help calm down the injured person or to assist in sleeping.

ADDITIONAL USES:
Super B and True Source vitamins have been used to promote healing of your skin.

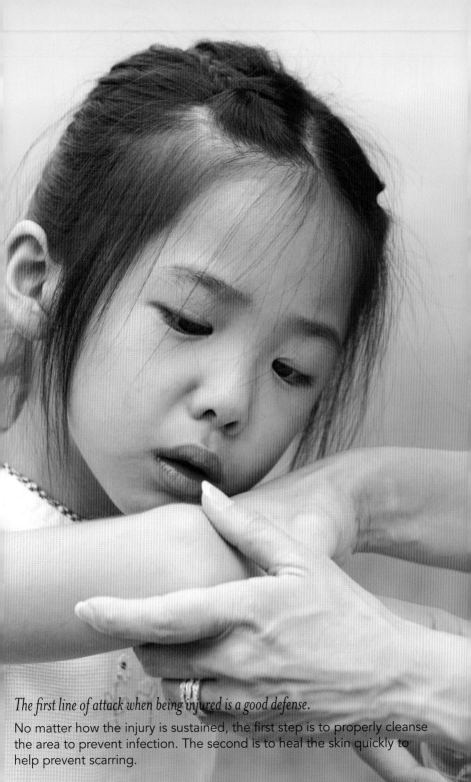

The first line of attack when being injured is a good defense.

No matter how the injury is sustained, the first step is to properly cleanse the area to prevent infection. The second is to heal the skin quickly to help prevent scarring.

DENTAL HEALTH

Healthy teeth and gums start with products that clean and protect without harsh chemicals. Discover the natural alternative to oral health with our essential oil-infused oral care products.

Young Living offers four different toothpastes for you and your family to choose from. Each one is a little different than the other and you may find that you, your partner, and your children may each like a different paste. Try them each out and see which one suits you better.

MAY WE ALSO SUGGEST...

TOPICAL:
Apply Thieves and Sacred Frankincense to gums 1-4 times a month to maintain good health. Thieves is also great for mild toothaches and infections. Brush daily with Dentarome™, Dentarome Plus™, Dentarome Ultra™ or KidScents™ Toothpaste.

DIFFUSING:
If visiting the dentist makes you or your children a little anxious, try diffusing Peace & Calming before your visit.

ADDITIONAL USES:
You can also try Alkalyme daily to maintain good pH balance in the body and support dental health. Before each meal, take an Essentialzymes-4™ capsule to aid digestion.

Your mouth is the gateway to your body and keeping a healthy mouth, including your teeth & gums, can affect your overall health.

Dental health goes beyond just your teeth and gums. Keep up with your dental hygiene and maintain the health of your teeth, gums, tongue and your throat - it will all help you insure good dental and overall health.

WHAT YOU WILL NEED...

Oil Blends	Single Oils	Also try...
• Peace and Calming	• Clove	• Balance Complete
• Thieves	• Lemon	• Essentialzyme
	• Peppermint	• Thieves™ Toothpaste
	• Sacred Frankincense	• Thieves™ Mouthwash

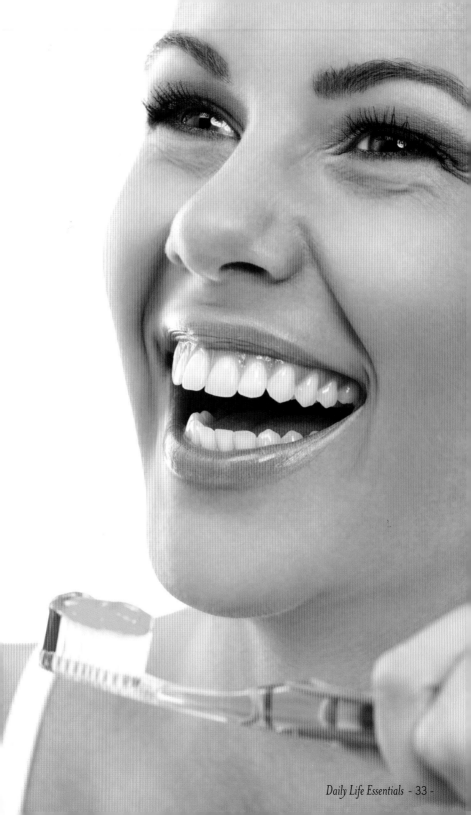

DIABETES

Diabetes is one of the leading causes of cardiovascular disease and premature death in Westernized countries. Diabetes causes low energy and persistently high blood glucose. Type I diabetes usually manifests by age 30 and is often considered to be genetic. Type II diabetes generally manifests later in life and may be linked to nutrition and dietary habits.

Diabetes is a disease in which your blood glucose levels, also known as blood sugar, are too high. Glucose comes from the foods we eat. Insulin is a hormone that helps the glucose get into your cells and create energy. With Type I diabetes, your body doesn't make its own insulin. In Type II diabetes, the more common type, the body makes insulin but doesn't use it well; the glucose stays in the blood instead of going into the cells.

WHAT YOU WILL NEED...

Oil Blends	Single Oils		Also try...
• EndoFlex	• Cassia	• Cypress	• Balance Complete
• DiGize	• Cinnamon	• Dill	• Essentialzymes-4
• Thieves	Bark	• Ocotea	• Mineral Essence
	• Clove	• Peppermint	
	• Coriander		

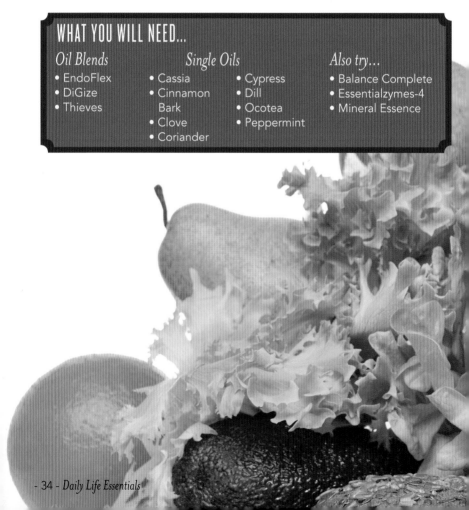

MAY WE ALSO SUGGEST...

TOPICAL:
Apply Dill and Cypress to the bottoms of the feet, 2 times daily.

DIFFUSING:
Diffuse Peppermint to clear the mind and reduce sugar cravings.

ADDITIONAL USES:
Try 4 drops of Ocotea and Cinnamon Bark under your tongue before meals. To help with sugar cravings, you can put 1 drop of Clove on the tip of your tongue. Dilute 50:50 with maple syrup.

You may not always have access to your essential oils if you're on the road. Try carrying Ocotea, Cassia or Cinnamon Bark with you no matter where you go. A drop of one of these oils under your tongue before eating can help regulate your blood sugar and help your body process the meal more effectively.

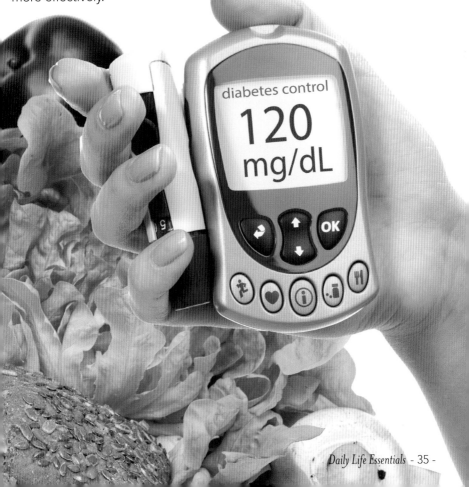

DIARRHEA

Essential oils can go a long way in alleviating some of the symptoms of diarrhea and promoting hydration.

Diarrhea Recipe:
- 4 drops Lemon
- 3 drops Mountain Savory
- 2 drops Wintergreen

As you're healing, even though you are thirsty, remember to drink water in small amounts at first to avoid nausea.

MAY WE ALSO SUGGEST...

TOPICAL:
Apply two drops of DiGize to the abdomen either neat or diluted. Start by applying often and then apply consistently every 2-4 hours for at least 24 hours after the diarrhea has subsided.

DIFFUSING:
You can use Peppermint to help settle the stomach.

ADDITIONAL USES:
A drop of Peppermint Vitality or Ginger Vitality in water until the symptoms have subsided. Follow that with one ounce of NingXia Red and a dropper of Mineral Essence every hour to help replace electrolytes in the body.

Diarrhea isn't just inconvenient, it can be painful and can lead to more serious illness.
No matter what causes diarrhea, the biggest threat to your body is dehydration. You can aid the healing process by keeping liquids in your body. Essential oils can help play a key role in maintaining hydration.

WHAT YOU WILL NEED...

Oil Blends	Single Oils		Also try...
• DiGize Vitality	• Clove	• Nutmeg	• Mineral Essence
• Ginger Vitality	• Lemon	• Peppermint	• NingXia Red
• Juva Flex	• Oregano	Vitality	
• Thieves	• Mountain Savory		

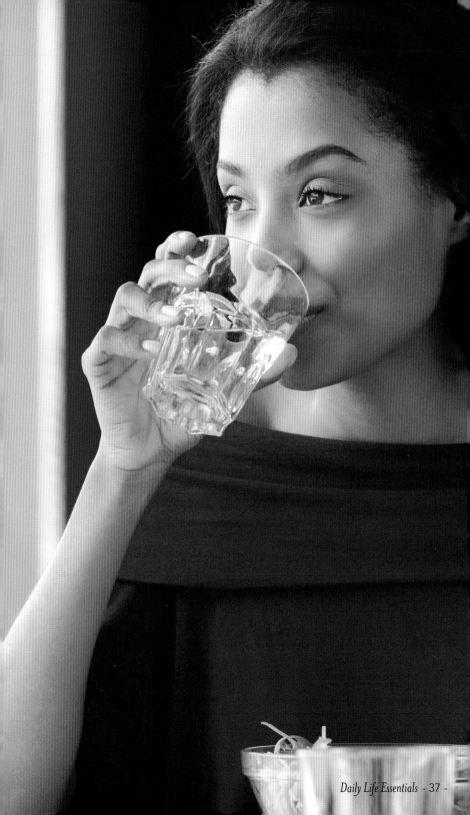

DIGESTION

A happy, balanced system is a healthy one. Whether it's a nutritive cleanse or an antioxidant-rich powder tablet, your system will thank you for all the benefits of our essential-oil-based products. Peppermint (Mentha piperita) has a strong, clean, fresh, minty aroma, and one of the oldest and most highly regarded herbs for soothing digestion. Studies have been conducted on Peppermint's role in improving taste and smell when inhaled which can aid digestion. DiGize™ is a dietary supplement that provides valuable aid for digestive concerns and helps support a healthy digestive system.* It is an ideal companion to the nutritional supplements ComforTone and JuvaTone®.

Problems with digestion can lead to more serious issues including ulcers. By maintaining balance in your digestive system, you can help lessen ulcers and other stomach ailments such as reflux and flatulence. Eat a diet rich in fruits and vegetables to help promote proper digestion.

WHAT YOU WILL NEED...

Oil Blends
- DiGize
- Peace & Calming
- Stress Away Roll-on

Single Oils
- Ginger
- Peppermint

Also try...
- Alkaline
- Carbozyme
- Digest & Cleanse™
- Detoxzymes
- Essentialzyme
- Life 5
- NingXia Red

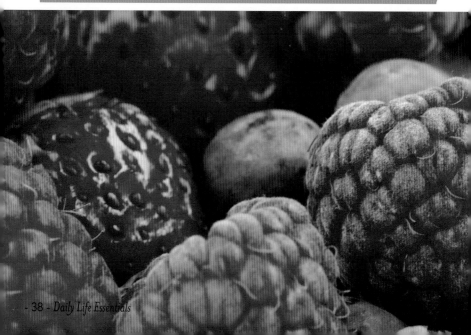

TOPICAL:
Apply two drops of DiGize, Ginger or Peppermint on the abdomen every day, more often if the problems are severe. Use Stress Away Roll-on to reduce the stress of chronic disorder.

DIFFUSING:
Diffuse Peace & Calming day and night to help reduce stress and lessen the strain on the digestive tract.

ADDITIONAL USES:
Take Essentialzyme-4 capsules with meals and a Life 5 capsule at night to support good digestion and healthy bowels. You can also take a Digest & Cleanse capsule between meals for extra support.

Digestive issues can be caused by myriad of behaviors and other common issues.

From an upset stomach after overeating or eating the wrong foods and experiencing tummy troubles, to more serious digestive disorders such as Crohn's Disease or IBS, eating properly and keeping your body healthy can make or break your digestive tract.

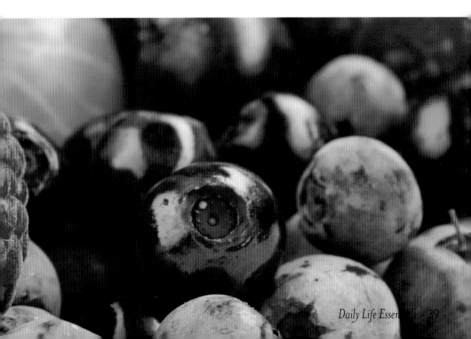

EARACHES

Earaches are most common in children but can affect a person of any age. An earache can be caused by many things, including dehydration, inflammation and an overabundance of pathogens. The pain can range from minor to completely debilitating. After you have treated your ear with the oils and the pain does not subside or gets worse, seek medical attention.

An earache can often lead to an ear infection. For that, you can try:
- Single Oils (Myrrh, Thyme, Wintergreen, Helichrysum)
- Blended Oils (ImmuPower, Melrose, Thieves, Purification

You can diffuse your choice of oils for 30 minutes every 4-6 hours or as desired. Try placing 2-3 drops of your favorite oil in your hands, cup your hands over your nose, and breathe in deeply through your nose. Repeat as often as you'd like throughout the day.

MAY WE ALSO SUGGEST...

TOPICAL:
Apply 2 drops of oil to a cotton swab (diluted 50/50 in warm olive oil) and swab around the opening of the ear - not in it. Put 2-3 drops of oil on piece of cotton and place carefully over the ear opening. Leave overnight.

DIFFUSING:
Lavender is a good choice for diffusing and is known for fighting germs and aiding in relaxation.

ADDITIONAL USES:
Try drinking 2 oz of NingXia Red and take an Inner Defense capsule during the day. Take a Life 5 capsule at night. Drinking water with Lemon or Citrus Fresh can aid in removing toxins from the body.

Ear pain can be very serious and can lead to an ear infection.
Treat your earache carefully.

You can apply PanAway (or another essential oil) gently around the ear to reduce swelling and assist with the pain. You always want to use a carrier oil and never put an essential oil directly into your ear!

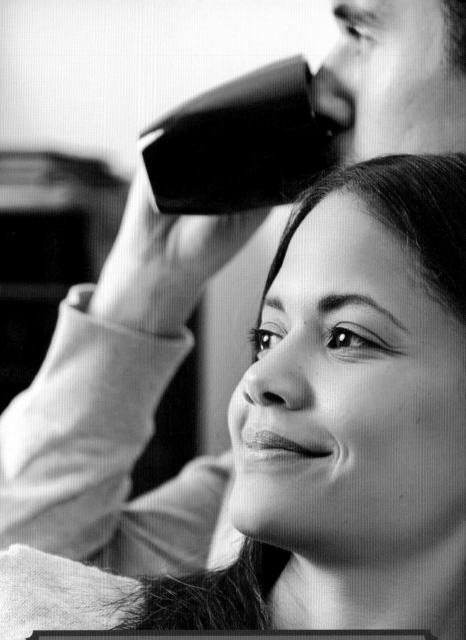

WHAT YOU WILL NEED...

Oil Blends
- Purification
- Pan Away
- ImmuPower
- Melrose

Single Oils
- Lavender
- Helichrysum
- Roman Chamomile
- Ravintsara
- Peppermint
- Eucalyptus
- Tea Tree (Melaleuca Alternifolia)

Also try...
- ImmuPro
- SuperC
- Super C Chewables

EMOTIONAL CONCERNS

Diffusing or directly inhaling essential oils can have an immediate, positive impact on mood. Your sense of smell (your olfactory system) is the only one of your senses that can have direct effects on the limbic region of the brain. Studies have even shown that some essential oils can stimulate blood flow and increase activity in the emotional regions of the brain.

To someone with depression, even the smallest daily task can be overwhelming. Try using one of the roll-on applicators (mix the oils ahead of time) to make the application process even easier. Nearly all the vitamins in the B group can play an active role in battling depression. Depression has been linked to deficiencies in B1 (thiamine) and B2 (riboflavin), while boosting an intake of B3 (niacinamide) has been shown to increase serotonin levels-which can also help fight depression. Serotonin is a neurotransmitter that helps communication between the two sides of our brain stay healthy. It is difficult to maintain balance if those two sides are not relaying messages clearly, so a lack of serotonin can definitely affect your mood.

MAY WE ALSO SUGGEST...

TOPICAL:
Apply Harmony™, White Angelica™, Valor and Joy 2-3 times a day over the heart, the wrists, and the feet.

DIFFUSING:
Peace & Calming can be used to help you relax. Citrus Fresh may be used to uplift the spirits.

ADDITIONAL USES:
Try drinking four ounces of NingXia Red and 3 OmegaGize[3] capsules, 3 times a day. SleepEssence capsules help at night and Essentialzyme capsules with each meal help with your digestive process.

Every year, more people report feelings of depression. It affects approximately 1 in 3 people across the country.

There are many medications that can help a person deal with depression, temporarily, but they are often accompanied by unpleasant side effects. There are many things you can change in your lifestyle that can have a dramatic effect on your mood and feeling of wellbeing, including healthy diet and increased physical activity.

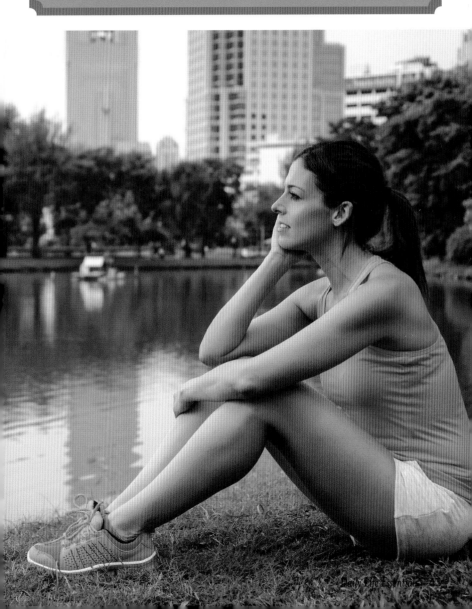

WHAT YOU WILL NEED...

Oil Blends
- Citrus Fresh
- Harmony
- Joy
- Peace & Calming
- Valor
- White Angelica

Single Oils
- Jasmine
- Frankincense
- Peppermint
- Ylang Ylang
- Rosemary
- Lemon
- Cedarwood

Also try...
- Essentialzyme
- NingXia Red
- OmegaGize[3]
- SleepEssence

Daily Life Essentials

EYES & SIGHT

You never appreciate what you've got until it's gone... and this is rarely more true than with your healthy eyes and good vision. It may start slowly with things far away becoming blurry, feeling like the magazine you're reading is too close, etc. But you can support the health and strength of your eyes in numerous ways. Vision problems can include a change in your vision, glaucoma, cataracts or even macular degeneration. The foods you eat, how much sleep you get, and how well you take care of your eyes can all factor into your eye health.

Carotenoids are natural pigments which are synthesized by plants and are responsible for the bright colors in fruits and vegetables, and they can be key to good vision. Power Meal, Balance Complete and NingXia Red are full of carotenoids. You can replace one meal a day or just add any of these as a snack. Blueberries are also a great source of potent antioxidants, such as anthocyanin, flavonoids and carotenoids. Blueberries have been found to support healthy neurological function and aid in maintaining normal eye health.

MAY WE ALSO SUGGEST...

TOPICAL:
Apply Frankincense, diluted, around the eyes and place Boswellia Wrinkle Cream on top.

DIFFUSING:
Peace & Calming and Lavender can both help you sleep at night. Restful sleep is imperative for good eye health.

ADDITIONAL USES:
NingXia Red, 3 OmegaGize[3] capsules and Longevity can be taken daily to support healthy vision.

WHAT YOU WILL NEED...

Oil Blends	Single Oils	Also try...
• Peace & Calming	• Clove (wet only)	• NingXia Red
• Longevity	• Frankincense	• Omega Blue
	• Lavender	• Longevity
	• Lemon (dry only)	• Carbozyme

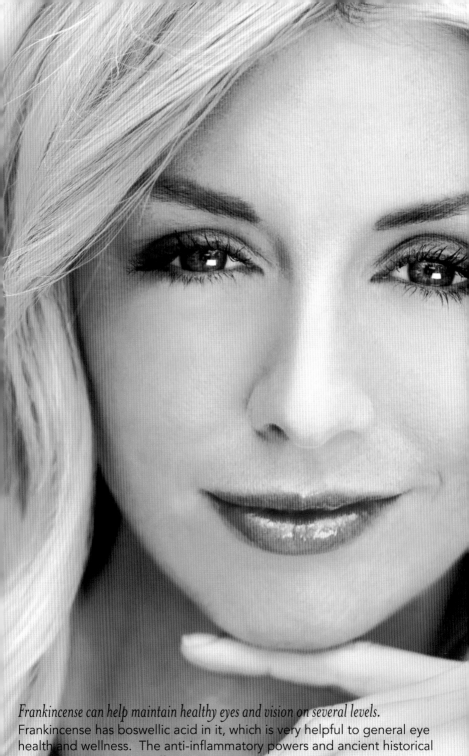

Frankincense can help maintain healthy eyes and vision on several levels.
Frankincense has boswellic acid in it, which is very helpful to general eye health and wellness. The anti-inflammatory powers and ancient historical uses demonstrate their effectiveness.

FATIGUE

Your body processes everything you eat and drink and changes it into energy that you can use. Although your body goes through the same process each time, it does not process everything in the same efficient, healthy manner. When we eat food that our body can not process, this can cause us to be sluggish and tired. This leads to sleepless nights, which can make you even more tired, and the cycle repeats and feeds on itself. When you are run down and exhausted, your body is more vulnerable to illness which can make you weaker and the cycle starts over again.

There are several things that add up to feeling fatigued. Hormone imbalances and mineral deficiencies can lower your energy. Natural progesterone for women and DHEA for men can be instrumental in helping battle the fatigue that comes with age and lower hormone levels. Pregnenolone is a precursor for both male and female hormones so both men and women can benefit from a pregnenolone supplement.

Physical fatigue, a general lack of energy, can be caused by a host of factors including adrenal imbalance and low thyroid activity. Digestion and colon issues can factor in as well so a liver and colon cleanse can help balance the digestive system and increase energy.

MAY WE ALSO SUGGEST...

TOPICAL:
Place a few drops of En-R-Gee on the back of your neck. You can also use Peppermint, Rosemary and Basil as a pick-me-up.

DIFFUSING:
Use Peppermint, Clarity™ or Lemon in your diffuser at home or office. These can help you retain focus and boost your energy levels, keeping your mind alert.

ADDITIONAL USES:
True Source vitamins and a Super B tablet can be taken before the biggest part of your day. NingXia Red and Multigreen capsules are a great replacement for caffeine and chocolate.

Building up your energy isn't just a daytime activity!
There are many things you can do during the day to help boost your energy - exercise, get some fresh air, eat healthy, etc. When taken at night, minerals can help promote a restful sleep which will provide more energy during the day.

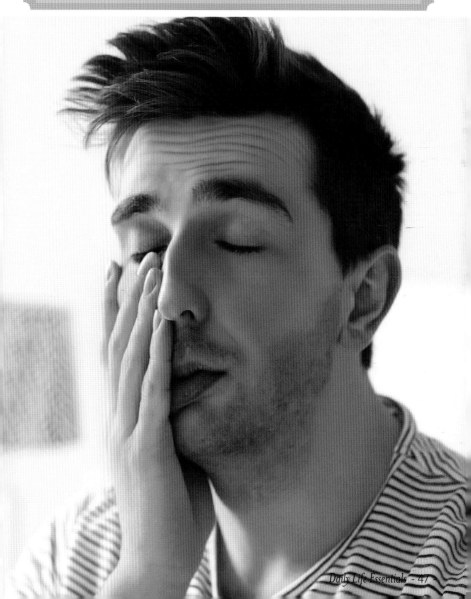

WHAT YOU WILL NEED...

Oil Blends
- Awaken
- Clarity
- En-R-Gee
- EndoFlex™
- Hope
- Motivation™
- Valor (& roll-on)

Single Oils
- Basil
- Cypress
- Eucalyptus Blue
- Dorado Azul
- Juniper
- Lemon
- Lemongrass
- Peppermint
- Rosemary
- Thyme

Also try...
- Life 5
- Multigreens
- NingXia Red
- Super B
- True Source

FEVERS

A good indication that an infection may be present in your body is a fever - an elevated body temperature. It is important to remember that if this fever increases or continues for a long period of time, you may want to seek medical attention right away. (Fevers over 104 degrees can lead to neurological damage.) Drugs can stop the fever immediately, but they also are stopping the body's alarm system. By using essential oils such as Oregano, Thyme, Mountain Savory, Thieves, Melrose and ImmuPower, you are adding powerful tools to your arsenal.

Fevers are one of the most powerful healing responses of the human body. Don't panic if your child has a low fever - sometimes that's a good sign that your child's body is doing what it's supposed to and fighting off a potential infection. Most bacteria and viruses live at body temperature so if the temperature is elevated, it creates an inhospitable environment for those "bugs" and they are killed off.

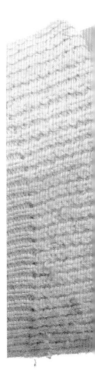

MAY WE ALSO SUGGEST...

TOPICAL:
Apply oils like Lemon, Peppermint and Lavender to the feet and back of the neck every 10-20 minutes until fever subsides.

DIFFUSING:
Diffuse Peace & Calming or Lavender to aid in peaceful and restful sleep.

ADDITIONAL USES:
You can also try one ounce of NingXia Red and a capsule of Inner Defense to support your body's natural defenses.

Your body can always use a little extra support when you're feeling under the weather.

When your body's temperature is elevated, it is called a fever, and it usually happens when your body is working harder than normal to fight off pathogens. Remember to stay hydrated (drink plenty of water) and don't eat a lot of heavy foods. This will help support your body as it fights.

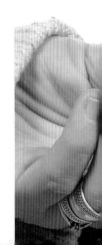

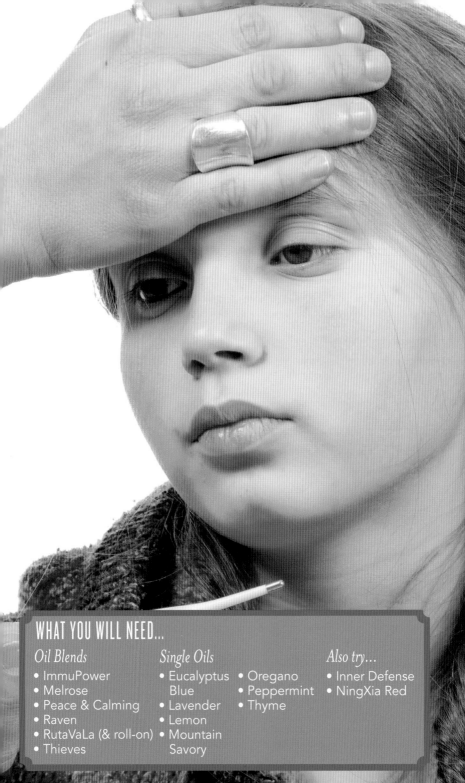

WHAT YOU WILL NEED...

Oil Blends
- ImmuPower
- Melrose
- Peace & Calming
- Raven
- RutaVaLa (& roll-on)
- Thieves

Single Oils
- Eucalyptus Blue
- Lavender
- Lemon
- Mountain Savory
- Oregano
- Peppermint
- Thyme

Also try...
- Inner Defense
- NingXia Red

FOCUS & CONCENTRATION

No matter what your day looks like (full of children, family, friends, work, deadlines, etc.) it is no doubt pulling you in several directions at once. Being able to focus fully on one thing at a time becomes a challenge - we are constantly getting interrupted and bombarded with things that beg for attention. Calming the nervous system and quieting the mind is key.

We can improve our focus and concentration by building our brain power, by giving it the food and care that it needs to best serve you. Brain Power is a powerful blend that can help give your brain a boost by using essential oils high in sesquiterpenes. You can use this to clarify your thoughts and develop greater focus. Try making a plan for your day, your week, and so forth. It is hard to function without a clear plan so by taking a few moments to organize your day, you can, in turn, organize your thoughts and allow a little more clarification.

MAY WE ALSO SUGGEST...

TOPICAL:
Use Clarity on the temples and back of neck and Brain Power can be applied to the big toes.

DIFFUSING:
When you need to concentrate, study or work for long periods of time, you can diffuse Peppermint.

ADDITIONAL USES:
Core Supplements, take NingXia Red daily. Feeding your brain with good nutrition can help you focus.

Don't overdo it - the mind works best in 20 minute increments!

Whether you're studying or working on long-term projects, give your brain a little break every 20 minutes. By walking away for just a minute or two, it allows your brain a break too. You'll be surprised at how much of a difference it can make.

WHAT YOU WILL NEED...

Oil Blends	Single Oils	Also try...
• Brain Power	• Peppermint	• Core Supplements
• Clarity		• NingXia Red

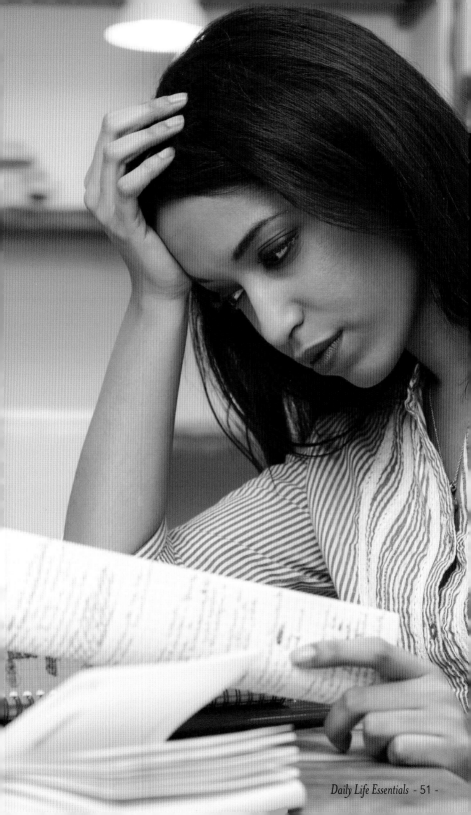

HAIR

Sulfur is the single most important mineral for maintaining the strength and integrity of the hair and hair follicle. We have a tendency to use products that can dry and damage our hair without realizing it. By using natural products, powered by essential oils, you can support your body's natural process of growing hair. When you take these products into the shower with you, be aware that a natural shampoo is oil based so if you want more foam and lather, add more water rather than more shampoo. By adding more shampoo, it adds more oil to the scalp and leaves hair limp.

Dry Scalp:
- 6 drops Cedarwood
- 2 drops Patchouli
- 2 drops Sandalwood or Geranium

Oily Scalp:
- 6 drops Peppermint
- 4 drops Lemon
- 2 drops Lavender
- 1 drop Peppermint

MAY WE ALSO SUGGEST...

TOPICAL:
Spring & Summer, use Lavender Mint Shampoo & Conditioner or if you have oil to normal hair. For normal to dry hair, or in fall & winter, use Copaiba Vanilla Shampoo and Conditioner.

DIFFUSING:
You can use a small amount of Animal Scents Ointment™ to dry hair overnight for deep conditioning.

ADDITIONAL USES:
Core Supplements, Sulfurzyme capsules and NingXia Red daily - feeding your body well will also help build beautiful, strong hair.

Have you looked into your hair care products lately? Perhaps we're too attentive to our hair.

Some of the most harmful products on the market are found in hair care products. We wash our hair so often and then use products for our scalp and hair... it could be doing more damage than we realize. Be aware of what kind of chemicals you're putting on your head.

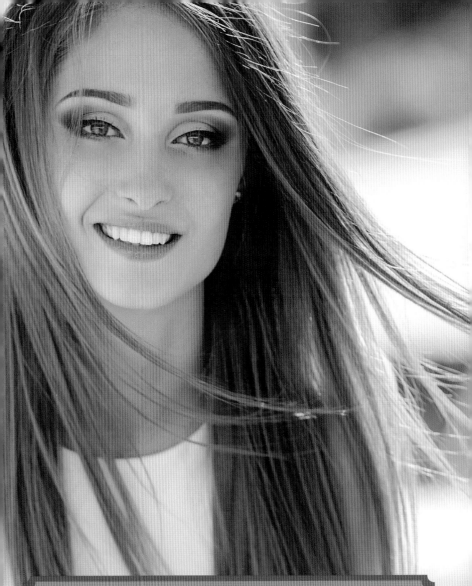

WHAT YOU WILL NEED...

Oil Blends
- Copaiba Vanilla Shampoo & Conditioner
- Lavender Mint Shampoo & Conditioner

Single Oils
- Cedarwood
- Clary Sage
- Cypress
- Lavender
- Melaleuca
- Orange
- Peppermint
- Rosemary

Also try...
- Copaiba Vanilla S&C
- Lavender Mint S&C
- Sulfurzyme

HEADACHES

Headaches are usually caused by hormone imbalances, circulatory problems, stress, sugar imbalance, misalignments and blood pressure issues. Essential oils can help promote circulation, reduce muscle spasms and decrease inflammatory response. You can also help prevent headaches by providing your body with healthy food, plenty of water, and getting plenty of exercise and rest.

General Headache #1:
- 4 drops Wintergreen
- 2 drops Lavender
- 3 drops German Chamomile
- 1 drop Clove
- 2 drops Copaiba

General Headache #2
- 4 drops Eucalyptus
- 6 drops Peppermint
- 2 drops Myrrh

Just for women:
Progessence Plus can help assist with the most common of headaches, those rooted in hormonal imbalances. The results can take time, hormone balancing can take weeks so don't get frustrated if you don't see immediate changes. Try for 8-10 weeks and see the difference.

MAY WE ALSO SUGGEST...

TOPICAL:
PanAway, Aroma Siez, or M-Grain™ to the temples and back of the neck. Try Prenolone® Plus Body Cream, Progessence Plus™ Serum

DIFFUSING:
Peppermint and Basil can be used during your headache. Also take a few minutes to lie down and breathe deeply.

ADDITIONAL USES:
BLM™ and Sulfurzyme capsules combined with 2 ounces of NingXia Red during the day, Super B at night.

---

*A headache can bring on the most debilitating pain –
unfortunately they're very common.*

Headaches is incredibly common, knowing the source of your headache can help you find a remedy. For example, the essential oil best suited for a nasal/sinus headache may not be the same oil best used for a stress or hormone imbalance headache.

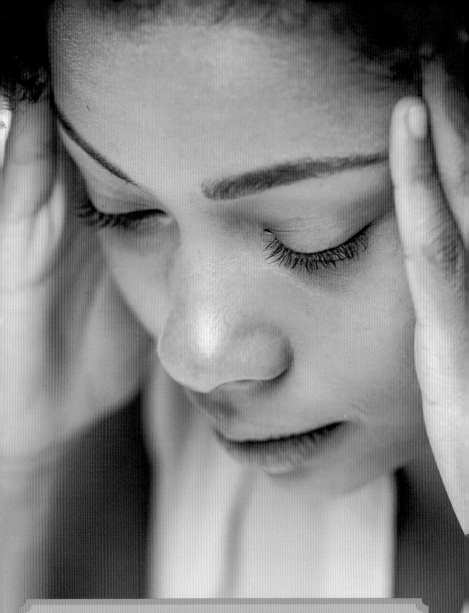

WHAT YOU WILL NEED...

Oil Blends
- Aroma Siez
- Brain Power
- Clarity
- M-Grain
- PanAway

Single Oils
- Basil
- Clove
- Copaiba
- Eucalyptus
- Idaho Tansy
- Peppermint
- Roman Chamomile
- Rosemary
- Raven

Also try...
- BLM
- NingXia Red
- Sulfurzyme
- Super B

IMMUNE SYSTEM SUPPORT

By now you've heard the buzz: antioxidants play a vital role in your health and help promote longevity. Give your body the power of antioxidants with our essential oil-infused support products.

One of the greatest advantages to an essential oil versus a lab-created medication or supplement is the ability to adapt. Just like your body and your immune system can adapt to the surroundings in an effort to maintain your health, the essential oils are based in nature and have the same attributes. A germ or bacteria that is becoming a "super bug" because it is building up a tolerance to all the medications we take can be fought with an essential oil that can adapt as well. Antibiotics and other medications are created to fight specific bugs and are not designed to change or adapt. If the bacteria gets ahead of the medication, you're fighting a losing battle. Medicinal plants have the ability to come back stronger and smarter.

WHAT YOU WILL NEED...

Oil Blends
- ImmuPower
- Longevity
- Melrose
- Purification
- Thieves

Also try...
- Inner Defense
- Life 5
- OmegaGize
- NingXia Red
- Super C

MAY WE ALSO SUGGEST...

TOPICAL:
Thieves can be applied to the bottom of the feet during fall & winter months; add Purification or Melrose to the bottom of the feet during spring and summer months.

DIFFUSING:
Thieves and Purification are your best defense to cleanse the air.

ADDITIONAL USES:
Inner Defense and Super C, drink NingXia Red during the day and take a Life 5 capsule at night.

A strong immune system is your most powerful defense against any illness.
The immune system is constantly changing and adapting to whatever pathogens are in the air. It tries to stay ahead of everything that attacks your body. Make it a daily focus to provide support for your immune system.

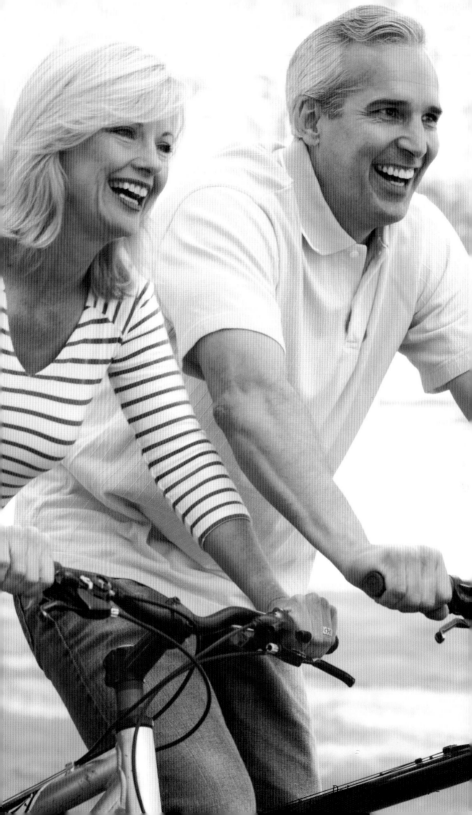

INSOMNIA

After age 40, sleep quality and quantity can deteriorate noticeably as melatonin production in the brain declines. Supplemental melatonin has been researched to dramatically improve sleep/wake cycles and combat age related insomnia. The fragrance of many essential oils can exert a powerful, calming effect on the mind through their influence on the limbic region of the brain (smell is the only way to directly affect that area). Lavender packs have long been used for infants, children and adults.

Insomnia Recipe
- 12 drops Orange
- 4 drops Dorado Azul
- 2 drops Roman Chamomile
- 8 drops Lavender
- 3 drops Valerian

WHAT YOU WILL NEED...

Oil Blends
- Peace & Calming
- RutaVaLa
- Sacred Mountain™
- Stress Away Roll-on
- Tranquil Roll-on

Single Oils
- Lavender
- Nutmeg
- Orange
- Sandalwood
- Valerian

Also try...
- ImmuPro
- Multigreens
- NingXia Red
- SleepEssence

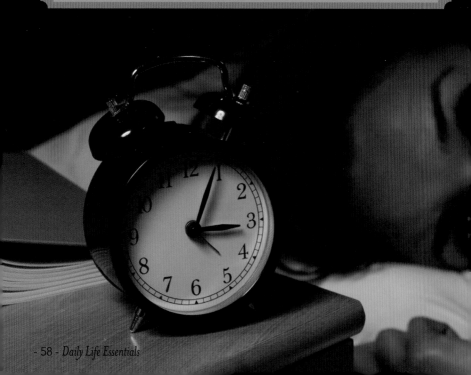

TOPICAL:
Lavender, Tranquil Roll-on, Peace & Calming Roll-on, RutaVaLa, or Valerian.

DIFFUSING:
Use your favorite calming oil - Lavender, Peace & Calming, Orange, Sacred Mountain, Stress Away Roll-on.

ADDITIONAL USES:
ImmuPro tablets or SleepEssence capsules. You can also use a drop of Valerian under your tongue.

Sleeplessness can be caused by a number of things and be quite hard to diagnose and overcome.

Whether you are stressed, sick, experiencing hormonal imbalance, or are depressed, sleeplessness can become chronic and actually lead to other health problems. Being able to sleep well is critical for good health and wellbeing.

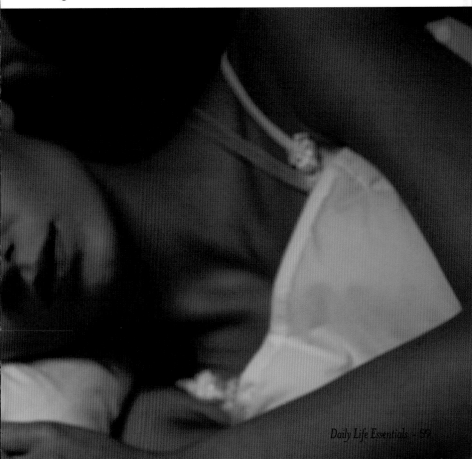

MEN'S HEALTH

As men age, their DHEA and testosterone levels decline. Conversely, levels of dihydrotestosterone (DHT) increase which contributes to prostate enlargement and hair loss. Men can directly benefit from pregnenolone creams as a way of jump-starting the sagging DHEA levels. Pregnenolone is the matter hormone from which all hormones are created.

Men often feel like they have the weight of the world on their shoulders; they allow the stress of family and work to come before their own health, to their own detriment. This can often lead to crises when left unchecked. There are ways to support men's health in natural and powerful ways:
  - Glucosamine can ease your joints.
  - Omega-3 protects your heart.
  - Vitamin E can slow effects of aging.
  - Folic Acid can support brain function.

MAY WE ALSO SUGGEST...

TOPICAL:
Shutran was developed specifically for men to help boost feelings of confidence and masculinity. It may be used topically as a cologne that appeals to both men and women.

DIFFUSING:
Idaho Blue Spruce has been formulated with high percentages of alpha-pinena and limonene and has a relaxing evergreen aroma. Diffuse each day for 30 minutes every 4-6 hours.

ADDITIONAL USES:
Clary Sage has been used to promote a calm and relaxing environment. Frankincense can be diffused or inhaled during meditation or it can be added to your favorite skin care product to enhance your complexion.

You are your own best caretaker! It is your responsibility to listen to your body and provide it adequate support.

Making small changes can affect your health in big ways - improving your longevity and strength. Start now taking a regimen of supplements, whole foods, and essential oils that may help protect you from ailments common to men.

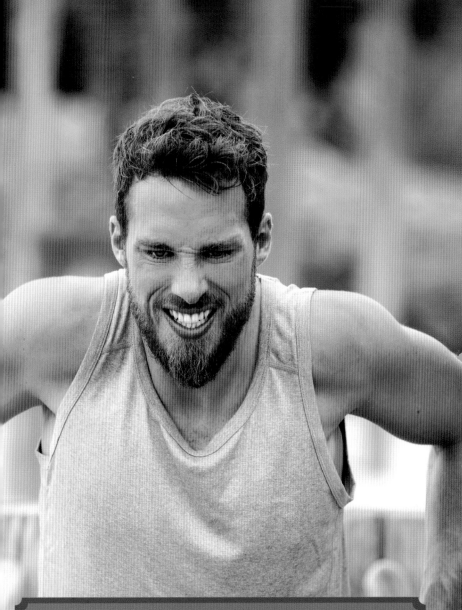

WHAT YOU WILL NEED...

Oil Blends
- Clary Sage
- En-R-Gee
- Mister
- Peace & Calming
- Shutran™
- Valor

Single Oils
- Fennel
- Geranium
- Rosemary
- Sage
- Frankincense

Also try...
- BLM
- Longevity
- NingXia Red
- Omega Blue
- Prostate Health™
- Super B

NUTRITION

Total health and wellness benefit everyone from age one to one hundred. The average diet of a typical person is grossly lacking in key nutrients. In addition to a lack of nutrients, food is being packed with preservatives, salts, sugars, and other fillers which can be addicting and usually contain empty calories. Adding a whole food supplement to your day is one way to break free from poor nutrition and increase a sluggish metabolism.

WHAT YOU WILL NEED...

Oil Blends
- Citrus Fresh
- Peace & Calming
- Thieves
- Valor

Single Oils
- Lemon
- Pine

Also try...
- Longevity
- NingXia Red
- Omega Blue
- Life 5
- True Source

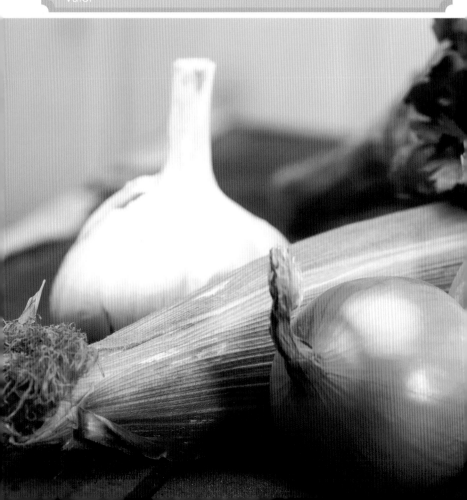

TOPICAL:
All essential oils can help with absorption of nutrients - try Thieves or Valor.

DIFFUSING:
Citrus Fresh, Peace & Calming, Pine can all be absorbed through inhaling as well as application and ingestion.

ADDITIONAL USES:
Try Core Supplements which include Longevity™, Omega Blue, Life 5, and True Source. NingXia Red is an excellent daily source of antioxidants.

Essential oils are natural companions of good nutrition.

Combine an essential oil with a whole food or a whole food supplement to create a homemade powerful health tool.

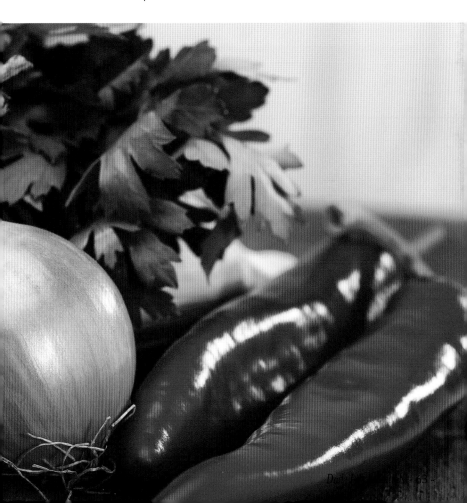

PAIN RELIEF

One of the most effective essential oils for blocking pain is Peppermint. Other essential oils have been shown to have unique pain-relieving properties including Helichrysum, Frankincense, Vetiver, Wintergreen and more.

PanAway is powerful in pain reduction. When applied on location or to the Vita Flex points on the feet, it can act within seconds. Alternate with Relieve It. These two blends are a great combination for deep-tissue pain as well as bone related pain. Deep Relief Roll-On is extremely helpful at home or work or when traveling.

Just because you're getting older doesn't mean you have to live with severe pain. By using essential oils directly on location or on the feet, you can pinpoint your pain spots and provide some relief. Additionally, you can use oils like Valor when getting acupuncture, doing yoga or receiving a massage- which can enhance your experience with these modalities.

WHAT YOU WILL NEED...

Oil Blends
- Aroma Siez
- Deep Relief Roll-on
- PanAway
- Peace & Calming
- Relieve it
- Valor

Single Oils
- Balsam Fir
- Copaiba
- Cypress
- Frankincense
- Helichrysum
- Lavender
- Spruce
- Wintergreen

Also try...
- BLM
- NingXia Red
- Sulfurzyme

MAY WE ALSO SUGGEST...

TOPICAL:
On location, apply PanAway, Aroma Siez, Deep Relief or Relieve It. For full-body massage you can use Ortho Ease or Ortho Sport.

DIFFUSING:
Peace & Calming or Lavender both work well. Tension and stress can make the pain seem unbearable so relaxation can be the first step to becoming pain free.

ADDITIONAL USES:
Drink NingXia Red and take BLM capsules daily.

Pain doesn't show up when it's most convenient for you – it can be present 24/7.
We can experience pain when we least expect it and, when it gets really intense, it can seem like there is no relief in sight. Fighting the root cause of the pain is the answer to relief. Essential oils can help fight the pain at the cellular level.

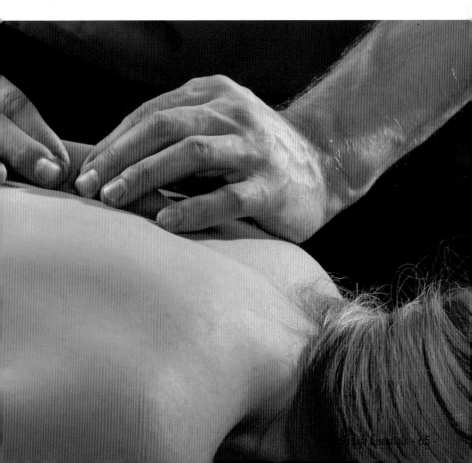

PREGNANCY

The more you know, the more you can do well by you and your baby. Try to eat mindfully. Be less reactionary. You can eat protein to help reduce sugar cravings. By staying active (be careful!), you can improve your posture. Surround yourself with goodness and positive energies (listen to those who are happy and have light, positive voices).

Labor Recipe (for use only after labor has started)
- 2 drops Helichrysum
- 2 drops Peppermint
- 2 drops Clary Sage
- 2 drops Fennel
- 5 drops Ylang Ylang

Optional Personal Care: Thieves Toothpaste and Mouthwash, Lavender Mint Conditioner & Shampoo, Lavender Bath Gel, Lip Balm and Lotion

MAY WE ALSO SUGGEST...

TOPICAL:
Your skin can be extra sensitive during pregnancy so no matter what oil you use, DILUTE it! Lemon, Lavender and Gentle Baby are commonly used.

DIFFUSING:
You can diffuse (or inhale directly) Ginger, Peppermint or DiGize to help alleviate nausea.

ADDITIONAL USES:
True Source vitamins (you may want to try KidScents® MightyVites™ as they may be easier on your stomach).

Know what you're getting into – you're protecting the health of two people now!

Using essential oils and other supplements while you're pregnant is not something you should do without weighing your options and consulting with your medical advisor and your partner.

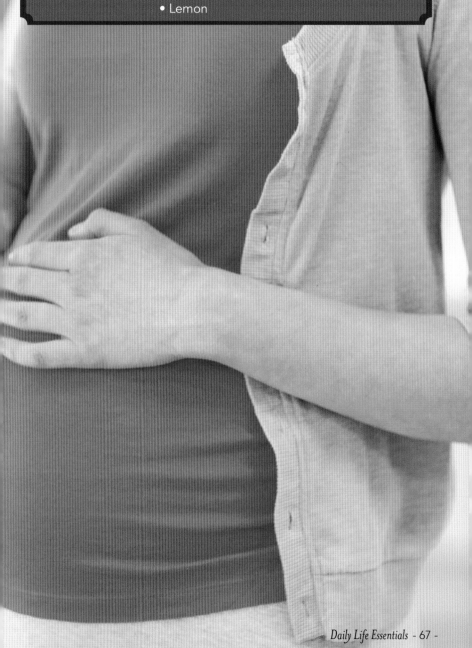

WHAT YOU WILL NEED...

Oil Blends
- DiGize
- Gentle Baby

Single Oils
- Ginger
- Peppermint
- Lavender
- Lemon

Also try...
- True Source
- KidScents MightyVites

RELAXATION & STRESS RELIEF

The world moves more quickly than ever and you can easily find yourself in the middle of a whirlwind of tasks, deadlines and obligations. When your task list for the day gets too long, all too often your precious "me time" is the first thing that is sacrificed.

For your mental and physical health, as well as your emotional balance, take a few moments to slow down and seek out the small moments of bliss. Rediscover tranquility with the beautiful scents of essential oils; they can be your natural solution to help relieve tension and troubles. Soul soothing oils like Lavender, Sandalwood and Spruce can help you overcome negativity and trauma and help keep you calm.

MAY WE ALSO SUGGEST...

TOPICAL:
Stress Away Roll-on can be applied to your pulse points. Alternate with Valor, Lavender and Peace & Calming. Nutmeg on your lower back can support your adrenals.

DIFFUSING:
Use your favorite calming oil including Lavender, Peace & Calming, Stress Away, Bergamot and Sacred Mountain.

ADDITIONAL USES:
Drink one ounce of NingXia Red and take 2 Multigreen capsules during the day to help keep your energy level up. This will help you sleep more restfully and allow you to recharge and be ready to face the next day.

WHAT YOU WILL NEED...

Oil Blends	Single Oils		Also try...
• Harmony	• Bergamot	• Lemon	• ImmuPro
• Joy	• Dill	• Nutmeg	• Multigreens
• Peace & Calming	• Idaho	• Rosemary	• NingXia Red
• Sacred Mountain	Balsam Fir	• Valerian	• SleepEssence
• Stress Away	• Lavender	• Vetiver	
(roll-on)			
• Valor			

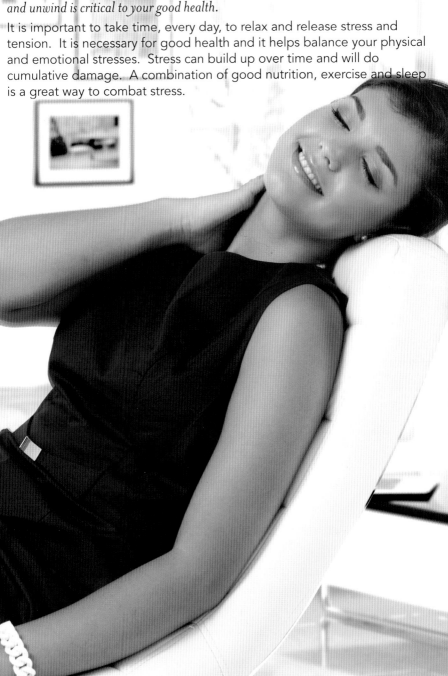

Whether it's a quiet walk in the park or a spa day with friends, taking time to relax and unwind is critical to your good health.

It is important to take time, every day, to relax and release stress and tension. It is necessary for good health and it helps balance your physical and emotional stresses. Stress can build up over time and will do cumulative damage. A combination of good nutrition, exercise and sleep is a great way to combat stress.

SEX DRIVE

Essential Oils can be very effective in stimulating your libido - increasing your sex drive. Enjoying an active sex life is an essential part of your general health and wellbeing. Our nutrition, including all the food we eat, can play a big part in helping us feel sexy. Some of the foods that can support your sexual appetite include pumpkin seeds, avocados, bee pollen and figs. Try using the supplements that include those ingredients - NingXia Red, Mineral Essence and Super Cal.

Just for Women:
- Ylang Ylang helps balance sexual emotion and sex drive concerns. Its aromatic influence elevates sexual energy and enhances relationships.
- Clary sage can help with the lack of sexual desire by regulating and balancing hormones.
- Nutmeg supports the nervous system to help overcome frigidity.

MAY WE ALSO SUGGEST...

TOPICAL:
Use Sandalwood, Jasmine, Rose, Ylang Ylang, Sensation™ or Live with Passion™ - apply to pulse points of both you and your partner (dilute with oil in sensitive areas).

DIFFUSING:
Jasmine or Sensation can be diffused to help "set the mood."

ADDITIONAL USES:
Longevity or OmegaGize[3] can be taken as directed. Drink NingXia Red for increased energy.

"It's not you, it's me... or maybe it's both of us."
Libido is more than just sex.

Libido is a combination of your mind and your body - your mental and emotional health come into play as much as your physical wellbeing. Sex drive can be affected by several factors including hormones, family, work, age, medications, stress and more.

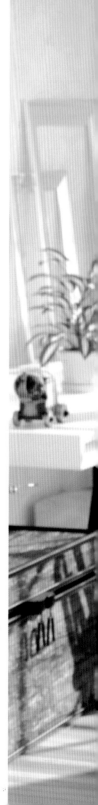

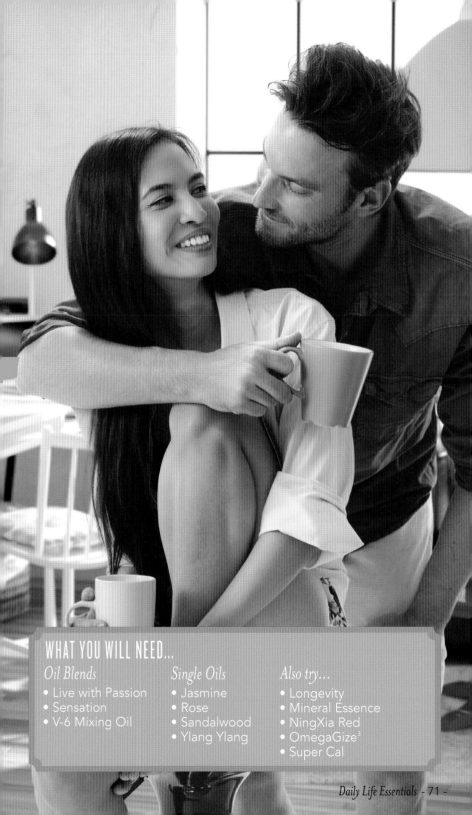

WHAT YOU WILL NEED...

Oil Blends
- Live with Passion
- Sensation
- V-6 Mixing Oil

Single Oils
- Jasmine
- Rose
- Sandalwood
- Ylang Ylang

Also try...
- Longevity
- Mineral Essence
- NingXia Red
- OmegaGize³
- Super Cal

SKIN CARE

The skin is the largest organ of your body. It is a major part of your immune system and can help regulate body temperature, protect you from outside pathogens and is an accurate indicator of your age and health. Take care of your skin and it will certainly take care of you.

Skin Rejuvenating: (mix with V-6™ Vegetable Oil Complex or unscented skin lotion)
- 6 drops Sandalwood
- 4 drops Geranium
- 3 drops Lavender
- 2 drops Sacred Frankincense

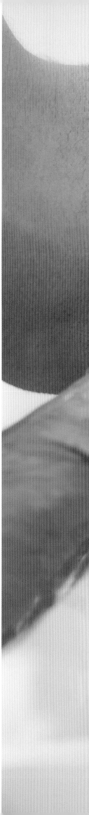

MAY WE ALSO SUGGEST...

TOPICAL:
ART Skin Care products are great for your face, including ART Skin Serum and Dry Skin Serum, ART Gentle Foaming Cleanser.

DIFFUSING:
Thieves and Purification can help kill airborne toxins that can harm the skin.

ADDITIONAL USES:
Three OmegaGize[3] capsules, 1 ounce of NingXia Red and 3 Sulfurzymes capsules daily.

Sometimes it's as simple as washing your face!

Wash your face every night - it's important to remove old makeup every night. Not only can they contain harmful chemicals but they can also trap air pollutants on your skin which can clog pores and cause damage to the skin's surface. Give your face a chance to repair itself while you sleep.

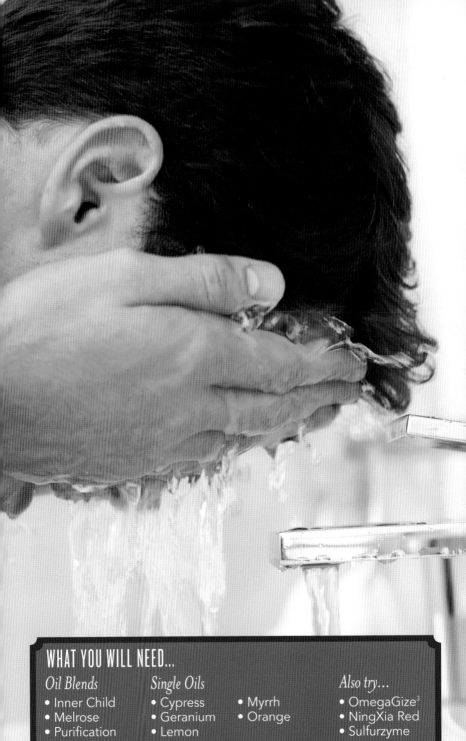

WHAT YOU WILL NEED...

Oil Blends
- Inner Child
- Melrose
- Purification
- Thieves

Single Oils
- Cypress
- Geranium
- Lemon
- Myrrh
- Orange

Also try...
- OmegaGize³
- NingXia Red
- Sulfurzyme

SORE THROAT

A sore throat can come from one of many sources - post nasal drip from a cold or allergies or swelling from an infection or a virus. If you ignore your sore throat, chances are it will take even longer for you to be back to health.

Sore Throat Recipe #1
- 2 drops Thyme
- 2 drops Cypress
- 1 drop Eucalyptus Blue (e.radiata)
- 1 drop Peppermint
- 1 drop Myrrh
- 1 tsp Honey

Sore Throat Recipe #2:
- 2 drops Eucalyptus (e. globulus)
- 5 drops Lemon
- 2 drops Wintergreen
- 1 drop Peppermint

WHAT YOU WILL NEED...

Oil Blends
- Melrose
- PanAway
- Raven
- Thieves

Single Oils
- Clove
- Cypress
- Eucalyptus Blue
- Frankincense
- Lavender
- Lemon
- Melaleuca
- Myrrh
- Oregano
- Peppermint
- Thyme

Also try...
- ImmuPro
- Life 5
- Super C
- Super Cal
- True Source

MAY WE ALSO SUGGEST...

TOPICAL:
Apply Lemon, Lavender and/or Thieves (diluted) to the outside of your throat. If pain persists, add diluted PanAway or Clove on top of the other oils.

DIFFUSING:
During the day diffuse Eucalyptus Blue and Melrose; during the night try Lavender.

ADDITIONAL USES:
Gargle with Thieves Mouthwash and suck on Thieves Lozenges throughout the day. Use Thieves Spray in the mouth and the back of the throat. Add Lemon and Frankincense to 1 ounce of NingXia Red.

A sore throat is one of the first indications that you're getting sick – it's a pain we all recognize and want to get rid of quickly.

Zinc has long been used to fight a sore throat because it is easy to use and because it is effective. Use a supplement that has Zinc in it including SuperCal, Super C and True Source.

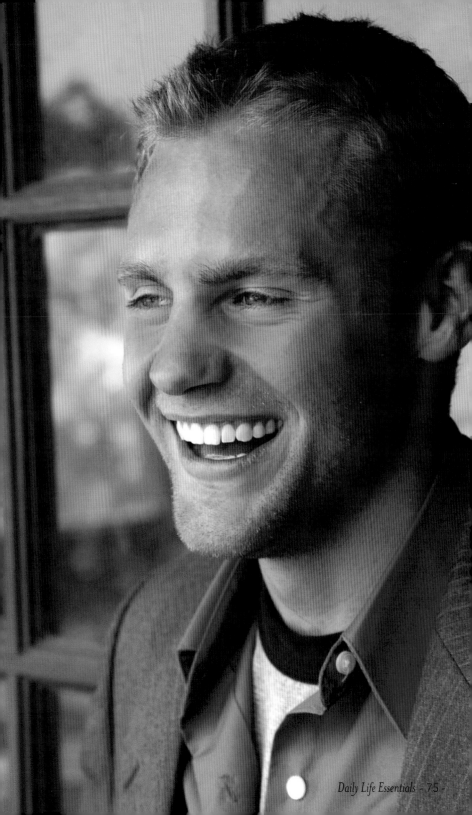

TUMMY TROUBLES

Sometimes when you're feeling sick to your stomach, the last thing you want to do is try to drink something. Try making an ice cube with a drop of essential oil inside - keep in mind that essential oils are very potent so you may want to dilute one drop in a large glass of water and then freeze it into small ice cubes. You may be able to handle sucking on an ice cube more easily than downing a glass of water and fighting to keep it down. You will still be able to benefit from the Peppermint. Ginger is one of the most widely used oils for nausea. It has been shown to improve digestion, calm nausea and support gastric health, just to name a few of its benefits.

Motion Sickness:
- 2 drops Peppermint
- 2 drops Patchouli
- 2 drops Ginger
- 5 drops V-6 Vegetable Oil

WHAT YOU WILL NEED...

Oil Blends
- DiGize
  (& Vitality)
- Juva Cleanse
- GLF

Single Oils
- Ginger
  (& Vitality)
- Nutmeg
- Ocotea

- Patchouli
- Peppermint
  (& Vitality)

Also try...
- Alkalime
- Detoxzyme
- Essentialzyme
- Digest & Cleanse

MAY WE ALSO SUGGEST...

TOPICAL:
Ginger, Peppermint or DiGize to back, feet, and abdomen.

DIFFUSING:
Either in a diffuser or directly inhale (put drops on your hands and cup hands over your nose) Ginger, Peppermint or DiGize.

ADDITIONAL USES:
Ginger Vitality, Peppermint Vitality or DiGize Vitality can all be added to a glass of water or add a drop or two to a capsule. Drink slowly to avoid more vomiting.

Our body has a great way of ridding itself of toxins – we get nauseated, or vomit. When we are digesting foods, our immune system slows down to send more power/energy to that system. By not overeating you allow your immune system to kick back into gear - listen to what your body is trying to tell you.

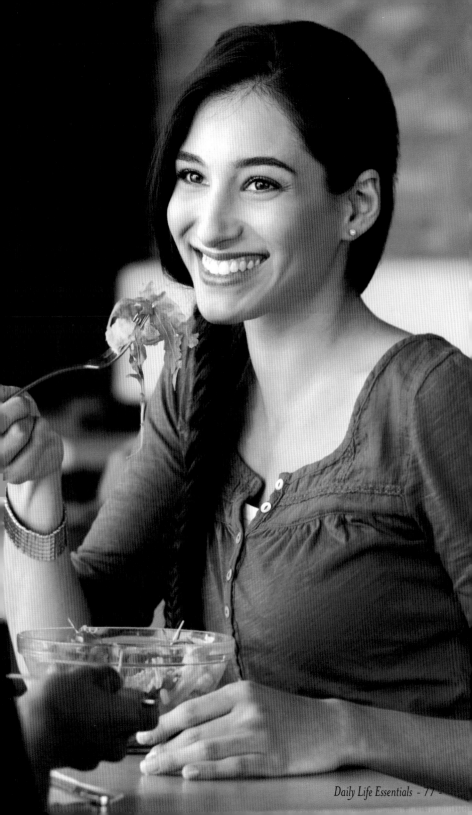

VIRUS

Viruses are responsible for everything from the common cold to AIDS, including the Ebola Virus, hemorrhagic fever, genital herpes, influenza, measles, smallpox, herpes, molluscum, chicken pox and shingles. Part of why a virus is so hard to kill (as opposed to a bacteria) is that it uses your body's own functioning system to help replicate itself - your body feeds it! You can help prevent viruses from spreading by maintaining a clean home and work space. Use Thieves Cleaner, Thieves Hand Purifier and Thieves Spray to help keep your living areas clean.

WHAT YOU WILL NEED...

Oil Blends	Single Oils		Also try...
• DiGize	• Eucalyptus	• Melissa	• Balance Complete
• Purification	Blue	• Oregano	• ImmuPro
• RC	• Lemon	• Rosemary	• Inner Defense
• Thieves	• Melaleuca	• Sandalwood	• Life 5
	Alternifolia	• Thyme	

MAY WE ALSO SUGGEST...

TOPICAL:
A drop or two of Melaleuca, Melissa, Rosemary, Thieves, Oregano, Sandalwood or Thyme can be applied to the feet and spine.

DIFFUSING:
Most effective germ fighters are Thieves, Lemon, Purification, RC, and Eucalyptus Blue.

ADDITIONAL USES:
NingXia Red and Inner Defense can help support your immune system. Sleep Essence can assist in good sleep patterns as well.

What is a Virus and what is doing to my body?
Your body will actually help fuel the Virus.

According to the Mayo Clinic, a virus is a little capsule, smaller than a single cell, that contains genetic material. To reproduce, the virus invades the cells of your body and uses your body's natural healthy cell process. The cells the virus invades (host cells) eventually die during this process.

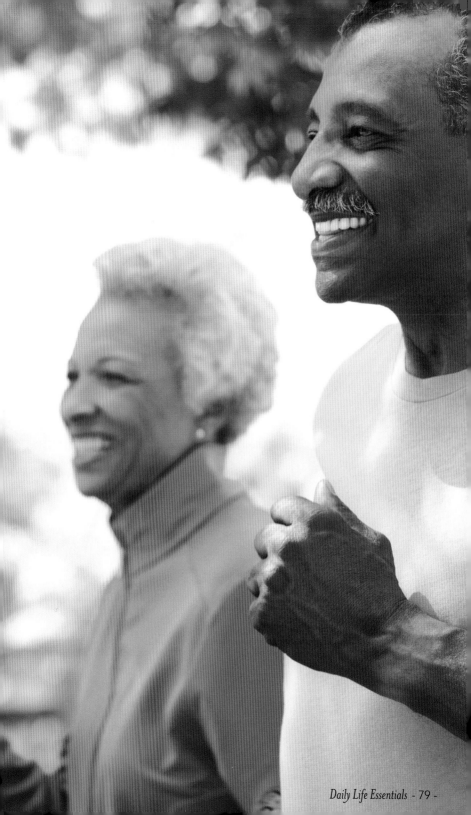

WEIGHT

Culture, age, diet, sleep, stress, sex, exercise and medications all factor in to your ability to maintain a healthy weight. If you're willing to create a formula and stick to it, you can absolutely reach and maintain your ideal weight.

Hormone treatments using natural progesterone (for women) and testosterone (for men) may be one of the most effective treatments for obesity. Progesterone levels can drop sharply after menopause and this can result in substantial weight gain, specifically around the thighs and hips. You can use transdermal creams to help replace declining progesterone, and this can result in a noticeably reduced body fat level.

Olfaction (smell) is the only sense that can have a direct effect on the limbic system so diffusing or directly inhaling essential oils can have positive impact on moods and appetites. Fragrance can penetrate the amygdala in the center of the brain so smelling pleasant aromas can help reduce your appetite.

WHAT YOU WILL NEED...

Oil Blends
- Slique Essence™
- Citrus Fresh

Single Oils
- Bergamot
- Bergamot Vitality
- Black Pepper
- Black Pepper Vitality
- Cypress
- Dill
- Dill Vitality

- Ginger
- Ginger Vitality
- Grapefruit
- Grapefruit Vitality
- Lemon
- Lemon Vitality
- Ocotea
- Orange
- Orange Vitality
- Peppermint
- Peppermint Vitality
- Tangerine
- Tangerine Vitality

Also try...
- Balance Complete
- Blue Agave
- Comfortone
- Digest & Cleanse
- Essentialzyme
- Essentialzymes-4
- 5 Day Cleanse
- Life 5
- Longevity
- Multigreens
- NingXia Red
- Omega Blue
- Slique Tea
- True Source

Feeling hungry? Maybe you should have some water.
You don't always need to eat when you're feeling hungry. Often times your cravings are not for food, but they are your body's way of telling you it needs something. Fill the void with hydration instead of empty calories. Need something crunchy instead? Try water rich foods like watermelon or cucumbers.

TOPICAL:
To help reduce cravings, try wearing Black Pepper with your favorite citrus oil (Grapefruit, Orange, Lemon, Tangerine or Bergamot). Dill can also be helpful when worn on the wrists.

DIFFUSING:
Place a little Citrus Fresh in your diffuser to fill your air with fruity goodness and help reduce cravings.

ADDITIONAL USES:
A little bit of your favorite Vitality citrus oils can be added to your water. Also check out Slique Essence - try a few drops in warm or cold drinks.

WOMEN'S HEALTH

Cortisol, a stress hormone, is one of the biggest adversaries of women's health. So many factors can attribute to your cortisol level - stress, age, lack of sleep, environmental and nutritional stresses, sedentary lifestyle, and caffeine can all drive cortisol to excessive levels. It inhibits the growth of good microflora in your intestines; (good bacteria) which can support your immune system, help create B vitamins, and increase the rate at which you absorb minerals like calcium, magnesium and iron. There are several indicators that the population of healthy bacteria is plummeting including more colds, sore throats, headaches, upset stomachs and even the overgrowth of dangerous bacteria and fungus like Candida.

WHAT YOU WILL NEED...

Oil Blends
- Believe
- En-R-Gee
- Gratitude
- M-Graine
- SclarEssence

Single Oils
- Basil
- Cedarwood
- Idaho Balsam Fir

Also try...
- CortiStop
- NingXia Red
- True Source
- Master Formula Hers

MAY WE ALSO SUGGEST...

TOPICAL:
Apply drops of Believe, En-R-Gee, or Gratitude to your pulse points. Progessence Plus can help balance your progesterone levels.

DIFFUSING:
Idaho Balsam Fir, Believe or Cedarwood (all oils and blends that originate in trees) can help support a woman's mind, body and soul.

ADDITIONAL USES:
True Source or Master Formula Hers can support better nutrition.

It's more than a feeling...
Managing the cortisol levels in your body can not only make you feel better but it can also affect how you LOOK. You may improve your hair and skin by reducing coffee and other sources of caffeine. Start drinking water with Vitality essential oils inside.

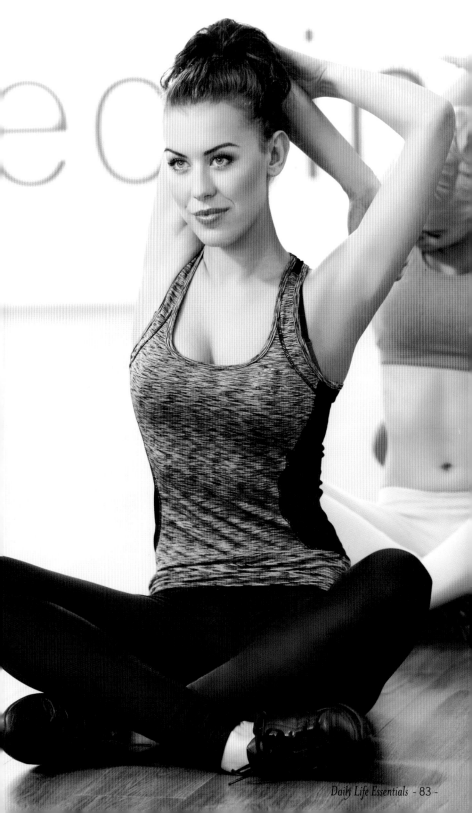